BEYOND CANCER

The Powerful

Effect of

Plant-Based

Eating

How to Adopt a Plant-Based Diet to Optimize
Cancer Survival and Long-Term Health

SALLY LIPSKY

A Note to Readers

This book is for informational purposes only and is not intended as a substitute for the advice and care of your health provider. As with all health advise, please consult with a doctor to make sure this program is appropriate for your individual circumstances. The author and publisher expressly disclaim responsibility for any adverse effects that may result from the use or application of the information contained in this book.

Dedication

For beloved Lara. And for Lani ("we must educate one another"), Lynn, and others who've demonstrated exceptional strength, courage, and grace fighting cancer. For patients who bravely participated in clinical trials to the benefit of others. And to Irene, my model of dignity and fortitude as a cancer patient and survivor.

To Dr. Joseph Kelley, Nora Lersch, and nurses and staff at Magee-Womens Hospital. I am forever grateful for their expertise, dedication, and compassionate care.

Finally, with deepest love and gratitude to Rick, Jennie, and Kylie.

Contents

Foreword

Sally Lipsky has written this book from a soulful place. She was diagnosed with late-stage ovarian cancer ten years ago but vowed that she would fight it. Not only has she fought the disease, she has conquered it, using food as medicine. Through extensive research, she discovered the power of plant-based nutrition. After healing herself, she decided to make it her life's work to bring this message to others.

Sally has a PhD in education and decades of experience teaching at the university level. It's not surprising she wrote this book from an educator's viewpoint, incorporating key elements of effective learning. Content is approachable and user friendly. When I sat down to read this book, I did not sit long. It was an easy read, which is a testament to the way Sally wrote and presented content.

Most impressive is Sally's humble, nonjudgmental way of communicating. I've been involved for quite a few years in communicating about benefits of plant-based nutrition and helping people change what they eat. I've learned that you cannot succeed in changing hearts, minds, and dietary practices by communicating in extreme or judgmental ways. Sally does not do this. She presents plant-based nutrition as being within reach of everyone.

I like that Sally advocates a balanced culinary philosophy consistent with what we have advocated in our organization. Plant-based eating should be joyful. Rather than dictating rules that create anxiety and disappointment, we want to focus on foods people can enjoy. There is only one important rule: do our best to consume whole, plant-based foods. Sally does a great job making this point in her book.

Two years ago, Sally left her successful academic career to focus on educating others about the power of plant-based nutrition. She made this decision because she knows from personal experience that plant-based nutrition can change lives. In addition, she is a compassionate woman who wants to change the world around this idea. As she shared with me, she believes societal change happens best in a grassroots way, from people helping people.

I hope you enjoy this book as much as I did. Follow Sally's example by sharing this important health message with people around you.

Nelson Campbell

Director of the film *PlantPure Nation*
Founder of PlantPure, Inc.

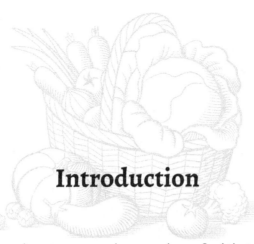

Introduction

*"Every day at every meal we can choose food that will
defend our bodies against the invasion of cancer."*
—David Servan-Schreiber, MD, PhD

Why I Wrote This Book

Like most cancer patients, I had little knowledge about the
powerful link between food choices and cancer. Only after diagnosis
did I begin learning about how certain foods can help prevent, fight,
and even reverse various cancers. This vital information did not come
from my physicians, nurses, hospital dietitians, or other health-care
practitioners. Nor did it come from often conflicting and confusing
headlines in mass media. I had to dig for this information. And I don't
want other cancer survivors to have to dig for the same information. I
write this book with cancer survivors, caregivers, and families in mind.
And for others seeking practical information about plant-based eating.

My Story

My life took an abrupt and shocking turn in August 2007.
A month after a clean bill of health from my gynecologist, I was
diagnosed with late-stage ovarian cancer. (Ovarian cancer often is
diagnosed at an advanced stage because of subtlety of symptoms
and lack of reliable screening tests.) I was stunned, especially since I
thought I maintained a healthy lifestyle. I exercised regularly and ate a
"good" diet, which included lots of dairy products, eggs, and poultry.

I immediately had surgery, followed by months of chemotherapy.

Most patients with my type of cancer experience recurrences within two years. Facing this alarming prognosis, and with two teenage daughters, I was determined to do whatever I could with dignity and grace. At this point, my doctor's visits were every 3 months. Before each visit, knowing I would receive test results, my anxiety would spiral upward. (To illustrate: before one appointment, I was so anxious a friend sent me Xanax tablets via overnight delivery!) Each time I received a report of normal test results, my anxiety instantly dissolved. Ahh—the joyous feeling of getting one's life back, at least for a few more months!

On Valentine's Day 2008, I officially was in remission (though still receiving treatment). My husband and I celebrated. However, I remained ever-vigilant about cancer's return. I considered cancer to be a ticking time bomb, ready to explode inside me at any time.

Not long after, I read an interview with David Servan-Schreiber, a doctor and neuroscientist who discovered he had a brain tumor at age 31. In his book, **Anticancer: A New Way of Life**, he describes the roles that food and nutrition—along with changes in lifestyle—have in keeping cancer away. This book opened my eyes to the relationship between foods and health. I'd eaten the traditional Western diet all my life, never knowing the connection between food and disease.

I began reading more and more. I learned how foods consumed on a day-to-day basis have an immediate and lasting impact on health and well-being. Hippocrates' words began to ring true: "Let food be thy medicine and medicine be thy food." Soon I realized I had a powerful tool—food—to help me fend off cancer recurrence. This knowledge provided a much-needed sense of control and empowerment.

I write this book to spread this sense of empowerment to other cancer patients and survivors. Fewer than 40% of women with advanced-stage ovarian cancer live five years after diagnosis. I'm extremely fortunate. A decade after my diagnosis, I remain cancer-free. I'm convinced a plant-based diet—as well as a lifestyle with family, friends, yoga, and much gratitude—keeps cancer at bay.

Unfortunately, this knowledge is not widespread in our health-care systems and cancer support organizations. Physicians receive little, if any, training in nutrition. And most hospital kitchens are focused on cheap, not healthy, food. Thus, individuals must take charge of what they eat.

Plant-based eating is now the norm for my family and me. With this book, I want to help make plant-centered eating the norm for you and your family.

This book introduces you to the whats, whys, and hows of plant-based eating. You'll learn what a plant-based diet consists of and why eating whole plant foods maximizes healing and health. Importantly, you'll learn how to incorporate plant-based eating into your daily routine. With real-life situations and convenience in mind, the book focuses on step-by-step change so that you can create new eating habits. You'll read personal tips from plant-based eaters, some of whom are cancer survivors.

Additionally, consider this book a path to the many experienced professionals and leaders in the field of plant-based nutrition. To you, the reader, I pass on a host of resources, including organizations, books, and online sites.

"Why Should We Believe You?"

Several years ago, I was giving a presentation on plant-based eating to a small group of people. We were discussing the confusing information in popular media about what is "healthy eating." A woman turned to me and asked, "Why should we believe you?" I replied, "Because I am not selling anything and am not profiting from my work with you."

With this book, I am selling something. However, I authored this book not to make money but to educate others, especially cancer survivors. I am donating book proceeds to several nonprofit organizations that promote research, information, and education about how plant-based eating can transform our collective health and well-being.

How to Get the Most from This Book

The book contains useful tools to make your dietary transition less overwhelming and substantially more successful:

Read chapters in order. In the first three chapters, I give basic information about what a plant-based diet is (and isn't). Also, I tell why eating plant food is so important for preventing, controlling, and even reversing cancer. In the following chapters, I describe how to put plant-based eating into action.

Complete chapter activities. You're more likely to form new habits if you try suggestions and reflect on what does and does not work for you. I encourage you to write or type your answers to activities. The process of writing helps to clarify thoughts. Plus, you are more apt to follow through with change when you can refer to what you wrote previously.

Use resources in chapter 12. This chapter lists people, publications, and organizations committed to educating and supporting your transition to plant-based eating.

Collaborate with another person. Ask a family member, friend, or caregiver to read the book with you. Work together to bounce ideas off each other, experiment with recipes, and provide support. A partner will help you follow through with intentions and make your food journey more enjoyable.

Remain dedicated. I am providing you with basic information and steps. You provide the commitment needed to create lifelong habits. I encourage you to put thought and effort into this potentially lifesaving shift.

Enjoy! Celebrate any and all changes you make to better your health. Focus on the self-satisfaction that comes from gaining knowledge and instilling simple yet significant changes. And be patient with yourself. Accept missteps and then move on!

Finally, I invite you to visit my website, *PlantBasedEatingHub.com.* You will find additional information and recipes, a discussion forum, and contact information. Feel free to email me with your questions and comments.

I hope you find this book to be an informative and useful tool in your journey toward long-term health.

Best regards,

Sally

STARTING ACTIVITY

Before beginning your journey into plant-based eating, complete these two items.

1. *What do you hope to gain from reading this book?* Jot down as many things as come to mind.

2. List foods you have eaten during the last 24 hours. Be as precise as possible about meals, snacks, and drinks you consumed. Keep this list handy. You will return to it in later chapters as you learn more and more about plant-based eating.

1

What Is Plant-Based Eating?

"There are virtually no nutrients in animal-based foods that are not better provided by plants."
—T. Colin Campbell, PhD

Plant-based eating means you are eating a variety of "whole plant foods." Whole plant foods include:

- **Grains**, such as barley, buckwheat, couscous, farro, oatmeal, quinoa, and rice
- **Vegetables**, such as broccoli, cabbage, carrots, corn, lettuces, onions, potatoes, and squash
- **Legumes**, such as beans, chickpeas, lentils, peas, and soybeans
- **Fruits**, such as apples, avocado, berries, citrus, and melons
- **Nuts** and **seeds**

The term "whole" refers to plant foods that are not highly processed. Examples are whole-grain rice as opposed to the processed rice in rice cakes. Or whole soybeans as opposed to the soy in protein powders. A plant-based diet consists of both cooked and raw foods. A plant-based diet does not contain animal-based foods: no beef, pork, poultry, seafood, eggs, or dairy.

Like plant-based eaters, vegans do not eat animal-based foods. However, a distinction is that vegans may be consuming many foods of little nutritional value. For instance, a person eating a diet of chips, cookies, snack foods, and so on, can be vegan. Whole, plant-based eating can be equated with a "healthy" vegan diet.

1

Eating Labels: What are the Differences?

→ Whole Foods, Plant-Based: no animal foods; minimally processed foods; minimal added fats, oils, and sugar
→ Vegan: no animal foods
→ Vegetarian: no meat, poultry, or seafood; yes to dairy; maybe eggs
→ Omnivore: yes to animal foods; yes to plant foods

Of note: Worldwide rates of chronic disease are highest with meat-eating populations and lowest with plant-based eaters

> Live longer by eating plants: Dan Buettner researched global cultures where people live the longest and with a high quality of life. Common among these communities are diets rich in vegetables, fruits, and whole grains and with minimal meat.[1]

Guidelines: Approximate Daily Calories

T. Colin Campbell, PhD, is a pioneering researcher in the field of plant-based nutrition.[2] He recommends the following daily distribution of calories for optimal health. All calories are from plant foods:

→ 80% complex carbohydrates
→ 10% protein
→ 10% fat

Don't be alarmed at these percentages. These numbers are an *approximation*. Once you get acquainted with the plant-based lifestyle, you'll see this approximation is not out of reach for you.

I certainly am not a purist when it comes to this guideline. As illustrated on page 7, when I examined what I ate during a day, my calories approximated these percentages. These numbers are a guide for food choices. You do not need to count calories or be preoccupied with balancing nutrients on a plant-based diet.

Complex vs. Simple Carbohydrates?

People usually are astonished that the bulk of recommended daily calories comes from complex carbohydrates. (I was!) There is widespread misinformation in the popular media about avoiding carbs. Carbohydrates are composed of starches, sugars, and fiber. There are important differences among types of carbohydrates. The following chart illustrates the superior health benefits of **complex carbohydrates** as compared to **simple carbohydrates**.

Complex Carbohydrates	Simple Carbohydrates
Examples: Multigrain bread, pasta, brown rice, oatmeal Beans, peas, lentils Potatoes, corn, broccoli, bell peppers, cabbage Whole fruits	Examples: Refined grains (as in most baked goods) Fruit juices Added sugars (table sugar, honey, syrup, etc.)
High starch content	Low starch content
Complex sugars	Simple sugars
High fiber	Low fiber
Digested slowly	Digested quickly
Absorbed slowly	Absorbed quickly
Slow release of energy	Quick release of energy
Slowly raises blood glucose levels	Quickly raises blood glucose levels
High amount of nutrients	Low amount of nutrients
High hunger satisfaction (stomach feels full)	Low hunger satisfaction

Complex carbohydrates provide needed fuel and energy to sustain you throughout your day. It's not that simple carbohydrates are "bad." Instead, the goal is to rely mainly on complex carbohydrates and to minimize simple carbohydrates in your diet. As you will discover in chapter 5, complex carbohydrates form the basis of plant-centered meals.

Plants Contain Protein

For an average adult, the recommended daily allowance of grams of protein equals 36% of body weight, as measured in pounds.[3]

For example, a person weighing 150 pounds (68 kilograms or 10.7 stones) needs about 54 grams of protein daily. Use this formula to complete the following activity.

REFLECTION ACTIVITY

What is 36% of your body weight, in pounds? (If converting, 1 pound = .45 kilograms or .07 stones.) Fill in the blank:

I need about_____ grams of protein/day.

Refer to the list of foods and drinks you consumed in the last 24 hours (page xiii). Approximately how many grams of protein did you consume? The US Department of Agriculture's National Nutrient Database will help you figure this out: https://ndb.nal.usda.gov/ndb/.[4] Open the website, type in the food item, and select from the listing. The nutritional information, including grams of protein, will be displayed. Do this for each food item you ate. Add the protein grams for your total. Fill in the blank:

I ate approximately_____ grams of protein for one day.

If you are similar to the vast majority of people, you ate more than the recommended amount of protein. Most adult women need about 40–50 grams of protein daily; adult men need about 50–60 grams. Even most vegans eat more protein than required.

> Average protein eaten daily:[5]
> Meat eaters = 105 grams
> Vegetarians = 90 grams
> Vegans = 70 grams

Note that all three types of eaters exceed the 54 grams of protein needed by a 150-lb. person.

However, not all protein sources are alike. Animal protein is associated with higher levels of disease, including heart disease, type 2 diabetes, autoimmune diseases, and cancers.

Where do plant-based eaters get their daily protein? The next chart illustrates the average amount of protein consumed from five plant food sources: grains, legumes, vegetables, nuts and seeds, and nondairy milk products. Use this as a reference when someone asks, "Where do you get your protein?" (And they will ask!) You can reply, "From whole grains, beans, spinach, seeds, almond milk," and so on.

Plant-Based Diet: Average Daily Protein

Type of food:	Grains	Legumes	Vege-tables	Nuts, Seeds	Non-dairy Milk, Yogurt
Average protein per serving	3 grams	7 grams	2 grams	5 grams	4 grams
Recommended servings per day[6]	5 or more	2	4 or more	1	--
Total protein for type of food	at least 15 grams	14 grams	at least 8 grams	5 grams	4 grams
Total daily protein	At least 46 grams daily				

You'll be eating enough protein on a plant-based diet. Simply put, don't worry about protein!

Plants Contain Fat

The body needs very little fat for optimal health. You get all needed fats from whole plant foods. It is not necessary to add fats or oils to your food. (More about oil-free cooking in chapter 5.) Any type of oil is a highly processed food item. For instance, one tablespoon of olive oil equals 120 calories. All the calories are from fat. Plus, one tablespoon of oil does not go far when cooking or baking. But for that same 120 calories, you can eat 25 whole green olives.

120 CALORIES

1 tablespoon olive oil vs. 25 whole green olives

Fiber:	✗	✓
Nutrients:	✗	✓
Fullness:	✗	✓

Importantly, a low-fat diet is associated with lower rates of various cancers and increased rates of survival. Keeping a healthy weight is important to protect your body from cancer. A plant-based diet is an excellent way to lose excess body weight and keep weight off. When you reduce added fats and cooking oils, you can eat more whole plant foods and you'll maintain a healthy weight.

Even if you are not concerned about losing weight, a low-fat diet tends to be healthiest. (If you want to add weight, I will discuss this in chapter 7.)

Plants Contain Calcium

There is calcium in multiple plant sources. Leafy greens, beans, chia seeds, soy yogurt, and nondairy milk all contain calcium. Plus, calcium from plants is better absorbed in your body than calcium from cow's milk. Importantly, casein, the protein in dairy products, stimulates production of insulin-like growth factor (IGF). IGF is linked to higher inflammation and cancer cell growth. Research indicates that consumption of animal dairy products is associated with hormonal cancers (breast, prostate, ovarian).[7]

> Cheese is the food most people do not want to give up. And for good reason. Cheese contains mild opiates that signal brain receptors—the same brain receptors as heroin and morphine.[8] Cheese is both addictive and unhealthy. It's high in saturated fat, cholesterol, salt, and chemicals. Chapter 6 has cheese substitutes.

Plants Contain Fiber

Fiber is found **only** in plant foods. There is no dietary fiber in animal foods. Fiber is vital to disease prevention. A diet low in fiber is linked to a host of diseases, including cancer. We do not consume enough fiber in modern society. Adult females should eat at least 25 grams and adult males at least 33 grams of fiber daily. A 2012 research study concluded that fewer than 3% of adults ate even the minimum amount of recommended fiber.[9]

> Note: When just starting to add fiber to meals, proceed slowly to avoid uncomfortable effects of too much fiber. And drink lots of water.

Example: nutritional value of food eaten by the author. To illustrate guidelines in this chapter (and to satisfy my curiosity), I computed nutritional information for the foods I ate in 24 hours.

Sally's Nutritional Profile for a Day

		Protein grams	Fiber grams	Calories total	% calories from fat
Breakfast	Pancakes with applesauce, berries	10	12	346	8%
	Coffee with oat milk	2	1	69	14%
Lunch	Yam stuffed with beans and salsa	7	8	206	1%
	Green salad, walnuts	5	3.5	148	63%
Dinner	Pasta, vegetables, teriyaki sauce	14.5	13.5	391	7%
	Fruit salad	1	3	99	5%
Snacks	Popcorn, air-popped	2	2.5	62	10%
	Oatmeal with banana and berries	7	11	214	9%
	Dark chocolate	1.5	2.5	115	56%
Sally's total:		50 grams	57 grams	1,650 cal.	19% fat
Recommended for average adult woman:		40–50	at least 25	1,600–2,000	10%

My protein intake and total calories were in the recommended range, and I had much higher fiber intake. Notice that 19% of my total calories were from fat. Most fat calories were from the walnuts on my lunch salad and my daily dose of dark chocolate.

CHAPTER REFLECTION ACTIVITY

Take a moment to think about what you learned in this chapter. Share your answers to these questions with a family member or friend.

1. *What is one piece of information that surprised you?*

2. *What is the most helpful thing you've learned thus far?*

3. *What is a burning question you have at this point?* Write it down.

You'll check back later to see if your question has been answered.

Optional activity. Use the *National Nutrient Database* to compute nutritional information for foods **you** ate in 24 hours.

2

Cancer and Food: Why Plant-Based Eating Is Vital

*"Can we eat to starve cancer? Yes, we can: What we
eat three times a day is our chemotherapy."*
—William W. Li, MD, Angiogenesis Foundation

Roberta is a 77-year-old breast cancer survivor. Her energy and joyfulness are infectious. I can't help smiling when in her company. She is an inspiration. I share her story with you:

I was shocked by my cancer diagnosis in 2008. I was teaching fitness classes and thought I ate healthily. I went to the library and searched the topic of cancer and food. I read books and online materials (and still do!). Plant-based eating has become a delicious and nutritious venture for me. My doctors are amazed that I'm in such great shape at my age. My cancer hasn't returned. My cholesterol is way down. And I have lots of energy and am never tired. I remain adamant about teaching plant-based eating to others. My advice to cancer survivors:

- *Be your own advocate, be proactive, and teach yourself.*

- *Care for your body as you care for your car and your home. Put the right fuel in your body. For your body to work well, eat nutritious plant foods.*

- *Be resilient. You can change, no matter how old you are!*

Link Between Food and Cancer[10]

- An estimated 30–80% of cancers are related to diet.
- Only 2–5% of cancers are considered hereditary.
- Cancer largely is a preventable lifestyle disease.
- Lifestyle changes, including diet, have an enormous impact on cancer development.
- Within weeks of beginning to eat a plant-based diet, the body's defense against cancer improves dramatically.
- A plant-based diet strengthens cancer survival.
- A plant-based diet helps reverse some cancers.

Anti-Cancer Elements in Plants

Plant foods are the most effective foods for protecting from and fighting off disease. The chart illustrates the superiority of whole plant foods. Note the similar levels of protein in plant and animal foods. However, plant-based foods significantly outshine animal foods in essential nutrients, including fiber.

Nutrient Composition of Plant and Animal-Based Foods
(per 500 calories of energy)

Nutrient	Plant-Based Foods*	Animal-Based Foods**
Cholesterol (mg)	---	137
Fat (g)	4	36
Protein (g)	33	34
β-Carotene (mcg)	29,919	17
Dietary Fiber (g)	31	---
Vitamin C (mg)	293	4
Folate (mcg)	1168	19
Vitamin E (mg ATE)	11	0.5
Iron (mg)	20	2
Magnesium (mg)	548	51
Calcium (mg)	545	252

Equal parts of tomatoes, spinach, lima beans, peas, potatoes
**Equal parts of beef, pork, chicken, whole milk*
With permission from T. Colin Campbell Center for Nutritional Studies

Plant foods (grains, legumes, vegetables, fruits, nuts, teas) contain *phytonutrients*. Phytonutrients help fight off diseases, including cancer. Here are reasons why phytonutrients help suppress cancer growth:

Plants are Anti-Inflammatory

Inflammation is the link between factors causing cancer and factors preventing it.[11] Chronic inflammation in the body can stimulate disease, including the growth of cancer cells. The following chart lists some sources that hinder inflammation and others that increase inflammation.

Lower Inflammation:

- legumes
- nuts
- flax seeds (*ground*)
- ginger
- cruciferous vegetables (*broccoli, kale, cauliflower, Brussels sprouts, cabbage*)
- black pepper
- curcumin (*active compound in turmeric*)
- chocolate, at least 70% cacao

Raise Inflammation:

- chicken
- cheese
- eggs
- red meat
- animal fats
- refined white flour
- sugar
- excessive stress
- feelings of helplessness and despair

Plants are High in Antioxidants

High-antioxidant foods help reduce inflammation in the body. Plant foods average **64 times more antioxidants** than do animal foods.[12] Sources of antioxidants include:

- apples and pears
- berries
- dark green vegetables (*broccoli, spinach, kale*)
- herbs (*such as basil, rosemary, parsley*)
- large-stone summer fruit (*nectarines, peaches, plums*)
- nuts
- lycopene (*in watermelon and cooked tomatoes*)
- soy
- sweet potatoes
- tea: white, green, oolong, black
- turmeric/cumin/yellow curry
- vitamin C (*in citrus and other fruits/vegetables*)

Plants Enhance the Immune System

Plants help fortify your natural defense system, warding off disease. A strong immune system can spot and eliminate abnormal cancer cells. Some sources of immune system enhancers are:

- cruciferous vegetables
(*broccoli, kale, cauliflower,
Brussels sprouts, cabbage*)
- garlic
- mushrooms
- onions
- turmeric/cumin/yellow curry

ACTIVITY

Refer to your list of foods and drinks consumed in 24 hours (page xiii). *How would you rate levels of anti-inflammatory, antioxidant, and immune-strengthening properties?* Give yourself a number from 1 to 5: ___

1	2	3	4	5
☹**very low**		☺**so-so**		☺**very high**

*If you are not happy with your score, don't worry!
You are going to change that soon.*

Animal Protein Fuels Cancer

How many times have you heard "sugar is the fuel of cancer"? Instead, it is protein in meat and dairy that energizes cancer cells. (This is not to say that refined sugar is healthy.) Substantial evidence, across decades and continents, demonstrates the link between animal-based protein and cancer. In his groundbreaking book **The China Study**, T. Colin Campbell writes about his early research. He observed that "nutrients from animal-based foods increased tumor development while nutrients from plant-based food decreased tumor development."[13] What powerful results! Unfortunately, these results have yet to be part of mainstream health-care policies and practice.

What about the estrogen in soy? Soy contains *phytoestrogen* (plant estrogen), which is different from animal estrogen. Soy can protect against cancer. And, like other plants, soy has antioxidant and anti-inflammatory properties. Populations eating soy products have lower rates of various cancers, including breast cancer.[14]

Food Transcends Genes

Do not think that "cancer is in my genes" and is therefore inevitable. Foods can turn on and turn off your "genetic switch." If you are genetically predisposed to cancer, this is another reason to adopt plant-based eating habits.

↑*ANIMAL* FOODS = CANCER *ON* ↑

↑ *PLANT* FOODS = CANCER *OFF* ↓

Fiber and Cancer

Dietary fiber is important because it helps eliminate carcinogens from your body. Fiber provides a natural way to "detoxify." And fiber is found only in plant foods. High-fiber diets are linked with lower rates of many cancers, including colorectal cancer.

What About Sugar?

We eat too much refined sugar in modern society. Excessive sugar is associated with physical and emotional health issues.

However, the American Institute of Cancer Research notes that "consuming small amounts of sugar as part of an overall healthful diet is fine."[15] Many plant-based practitioners and organizations take a similar stand. I recall Dr. John McDougall[16] saying if you want to sprinkle sugar on your oatmeal, go for it! It is the eggs, bacon, and buttered toast you should avoid.

A problem with refined sugars is that our taste buds become accustomed to extreme sweetness. (Refined sweeteners include table sugar, honey, syrups, and so on.) It is wise to use sweeteners sparingly. Instead, make use of bananas, applesauce, dates, fruits, and other natural sweeteners.

Healthy Weight

Obesity is linked to many cancers. Excess body fat creates a storehouse for carcinogens. If you are concerned about excess weight, a whole food, plant-based diet is the most effective way to lose and keep off excess pounds. Why? Because you can eat a variety of foods that are filling, satisfying, and energizing—not to mention high in fiber and low in fat.[17]

Marty is a nurse. Here is her story:

In 2009, I had advanced-stage colon cancer that had spread into my abdomen and lymph nodes. In hindsight, I shouldn't have been surprised. I was vastly overweight (I'd been on various diets all my life), had hypertension, and chronic constipation. With a hectic, stressful schedule, I relied on fast food and junk food. I had surgery and chemotherapy. At one visit, I asked my oncologist if I could do anything to prevent cancer recurrence. He suggested PCRM's "Food for Life" classes at a local hospital [see chapter 12 resources]. *There I learned about plant-based eating. I was surprised how delicious the food was. I love to cook and began to fully embrace plant-based recipes. By 2013, I'd lost much weight, gotten off blood pressure medication, and completed a sprint triathlon! I never felt better. However...* [you'll read more about Marty in a later chapter].

REFLECTION ACTIVITY

1. *What is the most significant information you learned in this chapter?*

2. *Are you still not convinced about the strong connection between food and cancer? Do you have questions about the topic? Or do you want to learn more?* I suggest these resources:

   Dr. T. Colin Campbell. *The China Study: Startling Implications for Diet, Weight Loss and Long-Term Health* and *Whole: Rethinking the Science of Nutrition.* Campbell details his early research and discovery linking animal protein and cancer development. He gives in-depth scientific analysis, including supporting information and illustrations regarding human cells and the physiology of cancer development. Also, he details why scientific and medical establishments shun the topic of food, nutrition, and health.

   Dr. Michael Greger. *How Not to Die: Discover the Foods Scientifically Proven to Prevent and Reverse Disease.* Greger provides a comprehensive look at the impact of diet on disease. Greger devotes several chapters to various cancers. His research is extensive. Also, NutritionFacts.org has many videos and blog postings on cancer topics.

   PCRM.org. The Cancer Project provides advocacy and information about cancer prevention and survival, focusing on the link between nutrition and cancer. Free seminars and podcasts, *The Cancer Survivor's Guide,* and other resources and classes are available online.

What Plant-Based Eating Is Not: Myths and Misconceptions

"The cure for cancer will not be found under the
microscope; it's on the dinner plate."
—Paul Stitt, author

Below is a list of common misunderstandings about plant-based eating. (Originally, I held most of these misconceptions.) Underneath each is an explanation of actual plant-based eating practice.

Myth: *Plant-based means a diet of only salads and "rabbit food."*

Reality: *No one can subsist on greens alone!* Remember, the foundation of a plant-based diet is complex carbohydrates (brown rice, oatmeal, whole grain pasta, potatoes, beans, lentils, and so on). These foods provide you with much-needed fuel and energy. Chapter 5 will give you guidelines for preparing meals.

Myth: *Plant-based eating consists mainly of raw—not cooked—vegetables.*

Reality: *Cooked foods, as well as raw, are part of plant-based eating.* In some cases, cooking boosts absorption of vital nutrients by the body. For instance, there is evidence showing that the cancer-fighting nutrients in steamed vegetables are absorbed better than those in raw vegetables. Dr. Michael

Greger explains that while "light steaming can partially destroy some nutrients, the absorption of the remaining fraction is so boosted that it may be even healthier than raw."[18] For some vegetables—such as celery, carrots, and green beans—antioxidant levels increase when cooked.[19] In summary, do not think that to maximize nutritional value, you should eat only raw vegetables.

Myth: *Plant-based eating means plain, bland-tasting dishes.*

Reality: *Plant-based eating can include your favorite dishes and cuisines.* Once you get familiar with basic ingredients and substitutions, you readily can adapt recipes to tastes. This includes lasagna, spaghetti, pizza, chili, tacos, stir-fries, burgers, macaroni and cheese, pancakes, and so on. You will eat delicious-tasting food while still maintaining a healthful, plant-centered plate.

Myth: *Plant-based eating is only for "tree-hugging hippies," not normal society.*

Reality: *Plant-based eating has been going mainstream.* Increasingly, health-care systems and even businesses recognize the tremendous health benefits and cost savings from plant-based diets. The Physicians Committee for Responsible Medicine (PCRM) took its employee wellness program to GEICO insurance company, where participants' physical health and emotional well-being improved dramatically.[20] Kaiser Permanente, a large US-based health-care provider, recommends plant-based diets to patients. Professional associations such as the American Diabetes Association, the American Institute Cancer Research, and the Academy of Nutrition and Dietetics recognize the benefits of plant-centered eating.

Myth: *Plant-based eating is expensive, especially since I must buy only organic produce.*

Reality: *On the contrary, plant-based eating can be quite inexpensive.* The cost of rice, potatoes, and beans is a fraction of the expense of steak, seafood, and chicken. Think of the traditional notion of inexpensive "peasant" foods. Peasant diets consisted largely of grains, potatoes, corn, and beans because workers couldn't afford meat. Nowadays, meat is affordable and universal. We are battling diseases of affluence resulting from overconsumption of animal foods.

Regarding organic produce: I abide by the Environment Working Group's annual list of items with the highest amount of pesticides. I try to buy organic for these items. (Chapter 6 explains more.) On the other hand, keep in mind that consuming a non-organic apple is healthier than eating that chunk of cheese or piece of chicken.

Myth: *Plant-based eating will take so much work; I'll have to cook from scratch.*

Reality: *No, you won't! As you will see in upcoming chapters, plant-based eating can be easy and convenient.* You can use frozen fruits and vegetables, packaged grains, jarred sauces, canned beans, and so on.

Myth: *With plant-based eating, I need to be concerned about getting enough protein.*

Reality: *You do not have to worry about eating enough protein—* see chapter 1. By eating a range of grains, starchy and non-starchy vegetables, legumes, and fruits, you'll get more than enough protein.

Myth: *With plant-based eating, I need to be concerned about vitamins, minerals, and other essential nutrients. I will need to take lots of supplements.*

Reality: *When eating a mixture of whole plant foods, you will be maximizing their nutritional values.* Nutrients in foods are not isolated from one another. As Dr. T. Colin Campbell states, "Think of plant food as working together, in harmony, to produce optimal levels of nutrition."[21] You don't need supplements. It is healthier and safer to EAT your vitamins and minerals.

Vitamin B12 is one vitamin to add via a supplement. The recommended dietary amount is 2.4 micrograms per day. (I take 1,000 micrograms twice a week.) Also, various juices, plant-based milks, cereals, breads, and other grain products are fortified with vitamin B12.

Myth: *With plant-based eating, I won't be able to eat out at restaurants, attend parties, or go to social events.*

Reality: *I enjoy eating out regularly, and so can you.* You'll have choices at fast food eateries and sit-down restaurants. Chapter 8 shows you how to be mindful of menus and selections. Chapter 9 offers suggestions for navigating social events and family holiday meals.

4

Food: New Perspectives and New Habits

"The only way to make sense out of change is to plunge into it, move with it, and join the dance."
—Alan Watts, author

There is much evidence that:

→ Our standard diet, centered on animal and processed foods, is fueling chronic diseases, including cancers;
→ A whole food, plant-based diet is the healthiest way to eat and increases life expectancy.

Nevertheless, knowing the extraordinary benefits of plant-centered eating often does not translate into actual practice. What you eat is part of your day-to-day habits, social interactions, and emotional responses. The food you consume is intertwined with your sense of self: family traditions, cultural identities, and societal norms. Thus, be aware that sustained change in your daily eating habits will not necessarily be easy or without bumps. However, it *will* be worth it.

Let's begin with several key elements of personal change.

Changing Your View of Food

What are your perspectives on food and eating? Before diagnosis of cancer, I regarded food as a way to quiet a growling stomach, a family responsibility, or a focal point for socializing or celebrating. I did not consider food to be "medicine" or healthy fuel for my body.

After cancer, that changed. The more I read and learn, the more I realize the absolute importance of food in healing and long-term health. Food provides what is equivalent to nourishing medicine.

#1 REFLECTION ACTIVITY

Before continuing this journey, think about how you view food. Consider the importance of food in your current lifestyle. Jot down your answers to the following questions.

1. *What is the role of food and eating for your:*

    · Family and cultural traditions:

    · Holidays and celebrations:

    · Social and work situations:

2. *What are your personal:*

    · Food preferences:

    · Food cravings:

Changing Your Behaviors

Several factors influence how successful an individual is when attempting new activities.

Motivation. The person wants to succeed and reach her goals. She pushes herself to keep going, even in the face of obstacles.

Persistence. The person does not let hurdles stop him. When problems arise, he seeks help and perseveres.

Personal support network. The person has at least one family member or close friend she can rely on for encouragement and support. She connects with individuals who are responsible and caring. Have you identified an individual to provide reassurance and support? (Hopefully, that person is reading the book along with you.)

Patience and practice. The person is patient and forgiving with himself. Trying out ideas and creating new habits takes time. Don't expect to master the full scope of plant-based eating immediately.

#2 REFLECTION ACTIVITY

What motivates you to want to change your eating habits? Why are you considering a plant-based diet? List as many reasons as come to mind. Share your reasons with a friend or family member.

Establish Your Mantra

Your mantra is a word or phrase that is personal and meaningful to you. A personal mantra is a great motivational tool to use as you move along in your plant-eating journey. You will repeat this mantra over and over again to yourself. Use it when you need to feel grounded and committed.

My mantra is "**I really, really, really don't want cancer to come back.**" I've used this phrase often over the years. It provides comfort and boosts my commitment to a plant-based lifestyle.

Refer to the previous reflection activity. Identify one reason that is most important to you. In other words, which one will resonate with you when facing personal uncertainties and challenges? Make this your mantra. Write it down for easy referral. Use it as often as needed.

Complete the phrase: **My mantra is:**

You are ready to begin putting plant-based eating into action!

5

Meal Prep: Breakfast, Lunch, and Dinner

"Scientific research shows that health benefits increase as the amount of food from animal sources in the diet decreases."
—Physicians Committee for Responsible Medicine

I do not like to cook. And I judge a recipe by its length; if it's long, I'm not using it. In other words, I place a high value on ease and convenience. So I was grateful to learn plant-centered meals can be prepared easily. This chapter provides guidance on how to make simple yet tasty plant-based meals.

Three Steps for Plant-Based Dishes

Creating a plant-based dish is like constructing a building—start with a solid foundation. For plant-based dishes, the foundation consists of complex carbohydrates. As described in chapter 1, complex carbohydrates provide much-needed fuel, energy, and fiber. Next, add vegetables and fruits to your foundation. Then, choose spices, sauces, and condiments to give your dish the desired flavor. For each step, select from a wide variety of food. A sample grocery list for the three steps starts on page 33.

Step 1: *Start with one or more complex carbohydrates.*

☐ whole grains (ex: rice, quinoa, couscous)

☐ starchy vegetables (ex: potatoes, corn, squash)

☐ legumes (ex: chickpeas, beans, lentils)

Step 2: *Add non-starchy vegetables and/or fruits.* (ex: peppers, broccoli, pineapple chunks).

Step 3: *Add spices, sauces, and condiments.*

Breakfast Examples

- Oatmeal + berries + cinnamon
- Oil-free sautéed hash brown potatoes with garlic, onions, peppers + fresh fruit
- Multigrain bagel + hummus + sliced tomatoes
- Toasted whole-grain bread + peanut butter + sliced apples
- Shredded wheat cereal + nondairy milk + fresh fruit
- Oatmeal + banana + spinach + frozen berries + flax seeds blended into a smoothie

Lunch and Dinner Examples

- Corn tortilla + smashed pinto beans + guacamole + shredded greens
- Multigrain roll + portobello mushroom burger + mustard + pickles
- Butternut squash bisque + peas + curry powder
- Baked potato topped with beans + corn + salsa
- Whole-grain pasta + marinara sauce + cannellini beans + fresh herbs + olives
- Rice noodles + peas + cherry tomatoes + Thai seasoning
- Brown rice topped with bean chili + tomatoes + chopped lettuce
- Pizza shell + tomato sauce + sweet peppers, onions, mushrooms, avocado + sprinkled nutritional yeast

Each of these dishes can be a stand-alone meal. Or eat it with soup, salad, fruit, or other side dishes. Photos of plant-based dishes from my kitchen are on pages 35-36.

TRY-IT-OUT ACTIVITY

Plan two dishes for the day. Review the previous lists of meal examples for ideas and fill in steps 1 thru 3, for breakfast and dinner.

Breakfast:	**Dinner:**
Step 1:	Step 1:
+	+
Step 2:	Step 2:
+	+
Step 3:	Step 3:

Prepare each dish, then, evaluate: *Did you like it? Would you repeat it? Would you make changes?*

Cooking Without Oil or Shortening

I have the most control over food I prepare at home. I do not use oil when cooking at home. Remember: there are no "healthy" oils, not even olive oil or coconut oil. Most people are accustomed to automatically adding oil when sautéing, roasting vegetables, or making salad dressings. You do not need oil in your dishes. When you stop adding oil, you will be amazed at how your taste buds change. You start to taste "real" food underneath the added oil. Here are tips for oil-free cooking and baking:

→ Sauté foods in water, vegetable broth, or a vinaigrette dressing. Add a tablespoon or two of liquid at a time.

→ Use nonstick, ceramic-coated, or copper cookware. I adore my copper frying pan. I cook even traditionally sticky foods, such as pancakes, without lubricating the pan.

→ Use silicone bakeware when roasting or baking in the oven. Or line a baking dish with parchment paper or a silicone pad to prevent sticking.

→ Make oil-free dressings. Vinegar or citrus-based dressings, with added herbs and spices, are easy to make. The secret to my vinaigrette dressing is lots of Dijon mustard. For creamier dressings, use tofu, avocados, or ground nuts, plus seasonings (recipes pages 90-91).

→ Substitute unsweetened applesauce, ripe bananas, mashed dates, and ground flax seeds when baking. (See oil-free Banana Oat Bars on page 95.)

TRY-IT-OUT ACTIVITY

Try sautéing without oil. Instead, use water, vegetable broth (preferably low-sodium), or an oil-free dressing. *How successful was this endeavor? Did you notice any differences? What changes will you make next time you try oil-free sautéing?*

Four Pillars of Convenience

I. Buy Frozen, Canned, Precut, and Prewashed

I rely heavily on frozen vegetables and fruits. Frozen produce is flash-frozen after harvesting. Therefore, it is as nutritious as fresh-picked. The nutritional value of frozen is higher than that of fresh if the fresh produce has sat for days in a truck or on a shelf. Buy frozen vegetables without added salt and sauces.

Canned legumes and vegetables also ease food preparation. (If salt is added, rinse content before using.) In addition, buy prepackaged condiments and spices. Jars of minced ginger and garlic are staples for me.

Another staple is packages of prewashed lettuces. Also, when traveling or in a time crunch, I buy precut, packaged vegetables to use in salads, stir-fries, or grilling.

For the ultimate convenience, buy frozen plant-based meals. Add extra vegetables and spices to suit your taste. (See *PlantPure Nation* entrees in chapter 12.)

II. Use Time-Saving Kitchen Equipment

Microwaves cook food quickly and make it easy to cook without added oil. Plus, microwave-cooked foods retain about 97% of their antioxidants.[18]

Crockpots or slow cookers are handy for one-pot meals, soups, and stews. Crockpots are great for cooking dry beans (recipe page 86). Also, crockpots make it easy to prepare oatmeal, rice, and other grains hours before a meal.

Blenders and food processors offer many conveniences. I have three blenders and use at least one almost daily. The first is a small blender that quickly dices and chops vegetables for soups, salads, and one-pot meals. As you'll read in chapter 7, diced or minced vegetables add nourishment to dishes: inside sandwiches, on top of flatbread or pizza, mixed in with grains, and more.

My second blender is larger and high-powered. This is my go-to tool for pureeing food and crushing ice. I use it for smoothies, creamy soups, velvety salad dressings and dips, nut butters, and sandwich spreads.

My third is a hand-held immersion blender. I use it for creamy soups with a bit of chunkiness.

III. Prepare One-Pot Meals

One-pot meals are an excellent way to add convenience. Make extra-large batches of soups, stews, and variations of three-step dishes. Freeze your leftovers in containers. You'll appreciate knowing a meal is ready after a quick reheat.

Jeff Novick developed a 10-minute meal plan that I recommend highly. (I've timed myself. If ingredients are nearby, it really does take 10 minutes or less.) Here is his formula for quick and tasty one-pot meals:

Jeff Novick's 10-Minute Meals
1. Start with packaged tomatoes (no salt; whole, diced, or strained)
2. Add:
   - canned beans (14 oz)
   - frozen vegetables (1 lb)
   - a grain, potatoes, or another starchy vegetable
   - spices and seasonings (premixed, salt-free)

Jeff says, "Change types of beans, veggies, starch, and seasonings to come up with a variety of fast, easy dishes!" His recipe for Curried Indian Potato Stew is on page 85. (*By permission: Jeff Novick, MS, RDN, www.JeffNovick.com*)

Furthermore, an extra-large salad can be a one-pot meal. Start with the customary greens, tomatoes, cucumbers, onions, and so on. Then, add grains, starchy vegetables, legumes, and even fruits. For example, add leftover barley, cut-up potatoes, roasted chickpeas, and orange slices.

Cold grain, bean, and potato salads are satisfying main dishes. Prepare them ahead of time and refrigerate until ready to eat. They are convenient for potluck and social events. Recipes for Quinoa Carrot Salad and Mediterranean Couscous Salad are on page 89.

TRY-IT-OUT ACTIVITY

Pick a one-pot meal to try. Look at the recipes in the addendum or search for a recipe in a cookbook or online site (see chapter 12 resources).

After cooking and tasting, answer these questions: *Would I prepare this dish again? Why or why not? How could I modify it to better suit my tastes?* [Write down changes so you remember for next time.]

IV. Use a Freezer

I refer to my friend Linda Jones as "the freezer queen." Here are her suggestions for freezing ingredients. You will need a supply of ice cube trays and storage bags or containers.

My Freezer = My Friend by Linda Jones

The freezer can make your cooking easier, quicker, and tastier. For liquids, freeze in ice cube trays. Then, put the frozen cubes in plastic freezer bags and label the bags with names and dates. I stock these items in my freezer:

- ☐ Salsa cubes: My husband likes his food spicy, so these come in handy. Add to stews, soups, and quick pasta dishes.

- ☐ Pasta sauce cubes: Use for smaller portions of pasta.

- ☐ Low-sodium vegetable broth cubes: Use to sauté veggies. When cooking a grain or pasta, add cubes to boost flavor.

- ☐ Nondairy milk cubes: Use when making small quantities of salad dressings or sauces.

- ☐ Chickpea or black bean burgers: Put uncooked patties on a baking sheet lined with parchment paper. Freeze. Place frozen patties in freezer bags. If patties are already cooked, cool first; then freeze.

- ☐ Cooked grains and pasta: Freeze in sandwich-sized bags. Use for quick add-ins to soups, stews, or salads.

- ☐ Nuts: Freeze in snack-sized bags. Use for grab-and-go snacks.

- ☐ Grated orange and lemon zest: Adds a punch of taste. Use at the end of cooking soups, stews, and vegetables.

- ☐ Sweet potatoes: Boil potatoes (keep on the nutritious skins). Cut into chunks and freeze. Add to salads, soups, or stews.

- ☐ Fresh herbs: Wash and dry the herbs. Freeze them in snack baggies. Add to dishes, such as hummus, cashew spread, dressings, and sauces.

TRY-IT-OUT ACTIVITY

Which of Linda's tips are useful? Put a check next to suggestions that you will try. *What other ingredients do you freeze?*

Desserts

Your desire for sweets will change on a plant-based diet. You'll notice that traditional desserts taste too sweet. To my taste buds, even desserts in many popular plant-based cookbooks contain too much sweetener. Yet I do have a sweet tooth. Here are several options for sweet treats:

- ☐ **Frozen fresh fruit**—berries, grapes, and bananas—offer a sweet, refreshing snack, especially during summer months. A favorite treat is frozen chunks of bananas rolled in unsweetened cacao powder. Also, blend frozen fruit in a high-powered blender for a delicious sorbet (page 94).

☐ **Ripe bananas** provide sweetness in baked goods and smoothies (page 94). Buy multiple bunches of bananas. When they get overly ripe, cut bananas into chunks, bag them, and store in freezer.

☐ **Unsweetened cacao or cocoa powder*** is a delicious ingredient for smoothies, cooked oatmeal, and baked goods. You can also add it to nondairy milk as a hot or cold drink. When buying sweetened chocolate, look for at least 70% cacao. The higher the cacao content, the higher the antioxidant value.

* Raw cacao is considered the purest form of chocolate. Cocoa powder is a more processed version. When buying cacao or cocoa powder, choose unsweetened.

TRY-IT-OUT ACTIVITY

Look at the dessert recipes in the addendum. Choose one to make. If none appeal to you, try a recipe in a cookbook or online site (see chapter 12). After tasting it, answer these questions:

Did it satisfy your sweet tooth? In what ways would you alter it? Would you change the amount or type of sweetener, or add chocolate chips, berries, nuts, or dried fruit?

Step 1: Examples of Complex Carbohydrates

Whole Grains

- ☐ amaranth
- ☐ barley
- ☐ breads (*pizza crust, rolls, tortillas*)
- ☐ buckwheat
- ☐ bulgur
- ☐ couscous
- ☐ cereal (*read labels carefully!*)
- ☐ farro
- ☐ freekeh
- ☐ millet
- ☐ oatmeal
- ☐ pasta
- ☐ quinoa
- ☐ rice (*brown or red, preferably*)
- ☐ rye
- ☐ spelt
- ☐ wheat berries

Starchy Vegetables

- ☐ corn
- ☐ peas
- ☐ potatoes
- ☐ pumpkin
- ☐ squash
- ☐ zucchini

Legumes

- ☐ beans (*black, butter, cannellini, kidney, navy, pinto, black-eyed peas, lima*)
- ☐ chickpeas
- ☐ lentils
- ☐ soybeans

Step 2: Examples of Non-Starchy Vegetables and Fruits

Non-starchy Vegetables

- ☐ asparagus
- ☐ beans (*green, yellow, purple*)
- ☐ broccoli
- ☐ Brussels sprouts
- ☐ cabbage
- ☐ carrots
- ☐ cauliflower
- ☐ celery
- ☐ cucumbers
- ☐ greens (*arugula, bok choy, broccoli, collards, kale, lettuce, mustard, spinach, sprouts*)
- ☐ mushrooms
- ☐ onions
- ☐ peppers
- ☐ tomatoes

Fruits

- ☐ apples
- ☐ avocado
- ☐ bananas
- ☐ berries
- ☐ citrus
- ☐ grapes
- ☐ mango
- ☐ melons
- ☐ papaya
- ☐ pears
- ☐ pineapple
- ☐ stone fruits (*nectarines, plums, peaches*)

Step 3: Examples of Condiments, Sauces, Seasonings, and Other Flavorings

- ☐ apple butter, unsweetened
- ☐ cacao/cocoa powder (*unsweetened*)
- ☐ dried fruit
- ☐ herbs (*basil, dill, mint, oregano, parsley*)
- ☐ hummus
- ☐ lemon/lime
- ☐ mustard/ketchup
- ☐ nutritional yeast*
- ☐ sauces (*barbecue, chili, curry, soy*)
- ☐ spices (*curry, garlic, ginger, paprika, turmeric*)
- ☐ tahini (*ground sesame seeds*)
- ☐ vinegar
- ☐ nuts and nut butters
- ☐ olives
- ☐ salad dressing
- ☐ salsa

* Nutritional yeast is an inactive yeast. It is yellow and flaky with a nutty, cheese-like flavor. It contains lots of nutrients, especially B vitamins. Uses for nutritional yeast include:
  - Sprinkle as a cheese substitute on pizza, pasta, baked potatoes
  - Add to batters when baking
  - Add to oatmeal and grains as they cook
  - Use as a binder in veggie burgers
  - Sprinkle on popcorn
  - Use in dairy-free sauces

Photos from Sally's Kitchen

Breakfast
    Oatmeal + sliced banana + frozen mixed berries + greens
    Whole-grain pancakes + jarred applesauce + frozen blueberries

Lunch/Dinner
    Baked sweet potato + black beans + frozen corn + chopped
green pepper + chopped green onions
    Prepared pizza crust + jarred pizza sauce + sliced onions, sweet
peppers, broccoli, asparagus
    Quinoa + frozen mixed veggies + cherry tomatoes + curry sauce,
over lettuce

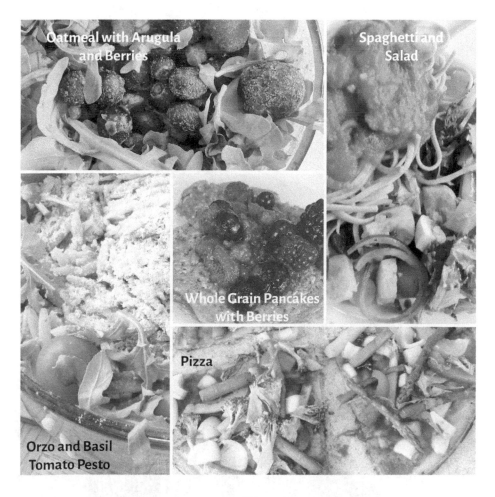

Rice noodles + frozen peas + cherry tomatoes + teriyaki dressing
Whole-grain spaghetti + ready-made, frozen seitan meatballs + jarred marinara sauce + side salad of raw vegetables with vinaigrette dressing
Orzo + arugula + cherry tomatoes + nutritional yeast topping

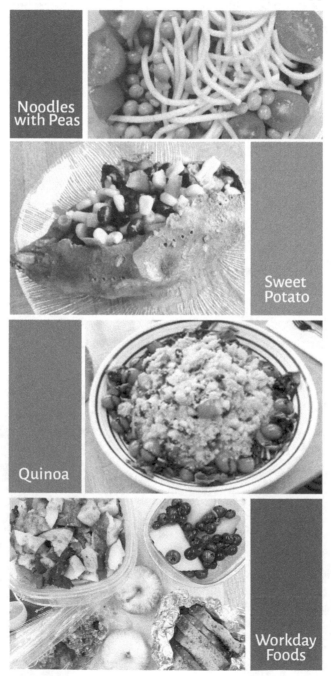

Shopping Tips

*"My #1 tip is stock frozen fruits and vegetables.
This is a tremendous time-saver."*
—Kylie L., longtime plant-based eater

Shopping for plant-based food items might seem confusing and overwhelming. However, it isn't.

Your local grocery store likely has basic ingredients and food items. It's not necessary to frequent food specialty stores. Here are my shopping suggestions:

Five Recommendations

Have a basic shopping list. For a comprehensive shopping guide, combine the list on page 38 with the lists on pages 33-34.

Buy fresh, frozen, canned, prepackaged, or bulk items. Choose what works for you!

Aim for a variety of colors. Eat a multicolored mixture of plant foods. The combinations will create a symphony of nutrients in your body. Do the food choices in your shopping cart reflect a range of colors?

Read labels on packaged items. Steer clear of highly processed food items, including supplemental powders for smoothies or juices. Also, be wary of items with many unfamiliar ingredients. Finally, be mindful of fat, added sugars, and sodium levels per serving.

Buy organic for certain produce. Organic produce generally is more expensive than conventionally grown. In addition, organic can be more difficult to find. I rely on the Environmental Working Group (EWG. org) for my guide as to which fruits and vegetables contain the most pesticides. EWG publishes an annual "Guide to Pesticides in Produce." The so-called "Dirty Dozen" have the highest levels of pesticides. Thin-skinned produce tends to be on this list. Examples are apples, berries, carrots, celery, cucumbers, lettuces, nectarines, peaches, spinach, sweet bell peppers, and tomatoes. If reasonable, buy organic for these items.

> Tip for washing produce: use one part white vinegar to three parts water. After a quick soaking, rinse in water.

Additional Grocery Items

Dairy Alternatives
☐ nondairy milk

☐ nondairy cheese

☐ nondairy yogurt

Meat-Like Items
☐ seitan

☐ tempeh

☐ tofu

☐ veggie burgers (*read ingredients, especially levels of salt/sodium and fats*)

Other
☐ applesauce (*unsweetened*)

☐ broth (*vegetable, low-sodium*)

☐ extracts (*coconut, peppermint, vanilla*)

☐ flour (*corn, wheat, rice*)

☐ pumpkin (*canned*)

☐ sweetener (*dry or liquid*)*

☐ teas/coffee

Dairy alternatives have become more commonplace.

Nondairy milks often are labeled as nondairy beverages. Soy and almond are the most common. Others include cashew, coconut, flax, hazelnut, hemp, oat, and rice milks.

If you are unfamiliar with nondairy milks, do a taste test to find which ones you enjoy. I keep three kinds in my house: oat milk for me (I like the sweet taste), soy for my daughter (she likes creaminess), and almond for baking. Also, you can make nondairy milk; there are plenty of online recipes.

Most packaged nondairy milks are fortified with calcium, vitamins, and minerals. They are sold in either refrigerated cartoons or shelf-stable packaging. When choosing a nondairy milk:

1. Sugar: look for one without added sugar.

2. Fat: some are especially high in fat. Coconut milk is high in saturated fats. If a recipe calls for coconut milk, I dilute it with water, buy the "light" variety, or use coconut water for flavoring.

Nondairy cheeses are made from nuts, vegetable oils, tapioca, soy protein, and similar ingredients. Most packaged brands are not a healthy food product. (And, to my taste, aren't appetizing.) They usually contain lots of oil. Also, some labeled as lactose-free contain casein, the protein in dairy linked to cancer cell growth. I suggest preparing your own. See recipes for easy nondairy cheeses on page 92.

Nondairy yogurts most often are soy, almond, or coconut based. Look for unsweetened.

Meat substitutes provide texture to dishes. They tend to be bland-tasting on their own but do absorb flavors of sauces and seasonings. They provide both protein and fiber, unlike "real" meat.

Seitan is made from wheat protein. I buy packaged seitan, though you can make seitan from scratch.

Tempeh is made from fermented soy with added grains. It has a slightly nutty flavor and chewy consistency.

Tofu is from soybeans and has a smooth texture. There are soft versions (good for sauces, dips, puddings) and firm versions (baking, stir-fries).

Add crumbled seitan, tempeh, or tofu to spaghetti sauces, barbecue sauces, sloppy joe sandwiches, and recipes calling for ground meat.

Premade, packaged **veggie burgers** are a convenient center to a meal. However, some contain dairy products (vegetarian, not vegan burgers). Also, many have high levels of fat and even higher levels of salt and sodium. You might want to make your own and freeze patties for later use.

> * Very few sweeteners have nutritional value. Date sugar (made from ground dates) and molasses have some nutritional value (Greger, 2009).[22] Erythritol is a "nontoxic, noncaloric" sweetener with some antioxidant activity (Greger, 2012).[23] Sweeteners with little to no nutritional value include maple syrup, honey, sugars (corn syrup, brown sugar, turbinado sugar, etc.), agave nectar, and brown rice syrup.

Avoid artificial sweeteners. Officially, they don't "appear to pose any health risks when used in moderation."[24] However, even stevia, a plant-derived sweetener, is not totally harmless.[25] I recommend consuming natural sweeteners.

TRY-IT-OUT ACTIVITY

Choose at least one plant-based food item that you are unfamiliar with. Examine the sample grocery lists on pages 33-34 and page 38 for the following:

→ Nondairy milk product

→ Meat-like item

→ Whole grain

→ Type of vegetable or leafy green

→ Type of legume or bean

Then, buy it and try it. *Will you add it to your basic grocery list?*

Economical Shopping

Plant-based eating can enhance not only health, but also finances. Plant foods (beans, lentils, grains, etc.) are much cheaper than meat, poultry, and seafood. If you're concerned about keeping grocery costs low, here are additional tips:

Off-label or generic brands. Supermarket chains often have their brand of everyday food items. These are lower priced than well-known brands.

Ethnic markets. Try Asian, Middle Eastern, Indian, Mexican, and other ethnic markets. They frequently have less expensive versions of staples such as grains, legumes, and spices and seasonings.

Discount stores. Dollar and discount stores often stock a surprising variety of packaged grains, canned legumes and vegetables, and seasonings and dressings.

Warehouse stores. Members-only stores, such as Sam's, BJ's, and Wholesale Club, stock fresh and shelf-stable grocery items. Costco Wholesale stores sell an increasing number of plant-based and organic foods: grains and pasta, fresh produce, nondairy milks, frozen berries and vegetables, fresh guacamole and salsa, and so on. If you are shopping for a family, it's hard to beat warehouse store prices. The downside is you must buy large sizes.

Bulk bins. Food in bulk bins can be cheaper than prepackaged. Health food markets, ethnic markets, and larger grocery stores often sell loose food items in bins.

Sale items. When you see a sale, stock up, especially with shelf-stable items. For example, at a local discount store I saw boxed oat milk at half the usual price. I bought all 25 on the shelf!

Online shopping. You can buy many items online, frequently for lower prices than in stores. See chapter 12 for online shopping sites.

TRY-IT-OUT ACTIVITY

Shop and explore! When you discover a store or website that's helpful or unique, let others know. Post your shopping experiences on *PlantBasedEatingHub.com*.

7

Making Food More Nourishing

"Use FOOD as your vitamins and minerals."
—Roberta W., plant-based eater and cancer survivor

Remember the examples of anti-inflammatory, antioxidant, immune system-enhancing foods in chapter 2? This chapter highlights ways to add these foods to your diet.

Popular media periodically hails a certain food as "the" healthy food item. However, there is no one food you must eat for health. For instance, if you don't like kale, that's okay—find another leafy green vegetable. The same goes for food allergies and sensitivities. If you get an allergic reaction to a food (such as nuts, soy, or wheat), enjoy plant-based eating without it. But certain plant foods are especially high in cancer-fighting nutrients. Make a point to eat these foods often.

Suggestions for Fortifying Your Meals

Alliums

Alliums include chives, garlic, leeks, shallots, and scallions. They are a family of vegetables known for immune-strengthening properties.

Suggestions for Adding Alliums

- ☐ Dressings and sauces
- ☐ Jarred sauces
- ☐ Stir fry
- ☐ Soups, stews, and casseroles

☐ Cold salads

☐ Ethnic cuisines (Chinese, Indian, Mexican, Thai, etc.)

Other suggestions?

Berries

Berries are chock full of antioxidants. Your daily dose might include acai berries, amla (Indian gooseberries), blackberries, blueberries, boysenberries, cherries, cranberries, goji berries, raspberries, strawberries, and the list goes on.

Suggestions for Adding Berries

☐ Cooked or cold cereals

☐ Salads

☐ Grain dishes

☐ Smoothies or sorbets

☐ Nut butter sandwiches, instead of jelly (i.e., peanut butter and "whole berry" sandwich)

☐ Sparkling water or iced tea

☐ Sauces and spreads (see Mixed Berries Jalapeno Chia Spread on page 91)

Other suggestions?

Cruciferous Vegetables and Dark, Leafy Greens

Cruciferous vegetables and dark, leafy greens have high nutritional value. They are an important addition to an anticancer diet. Eat at least one serving daily. Examples are arugula, beet greens, bok choy, broccoli, Brussels sprouts, cabbage, chard, collard greens, kale, various lettuces, mustard greens, spinach, and sprouts.

Note: Make your greens convenient to eat. For instance, my husband is even less ambitious than I am about food preparation. I've created a "salad bin" in our refrigerator. The bin that used to hold packages of ingredients now holds an oversized mixed salad. I throw in a container of prewashed lettuce and add sliced cucumbers, onions, carrots, beets, etc. Now my husband can reach in and grab a handful of salad.

Suggestions for Adding Cruciferous Vegetables and Leafy Greens

- ☐ Maximize absorption of nutrients by eating greens with a source of plant-based fat (avocado, whole olives, walnuts, seeds)[26]

- ☐ Breakfast—in oatmeal or another grain, tofu stir-fry, morning smoothie, or on a bagel spread with nut butter

- ☐ Lunch and dinner—in sandwiches, wraps, stir-fry, soups, tacos, burritos, pasta, grain dishes, and on pizza

Other suggestions?

Flax Seeds

Flax seeds offer a rich source of anti-inflammatory omega-3 fatty acids. Flax is composed of lignans. Lignans are fiber-rich compounds with powerful anticancer qualities. Grind flax seeds to maximize absorption and effectiveness. Store ground seeds in the refrigerator.

Suggestions for Adding Flax Seed

- ☐ Morning cereal
- ☐ Salad dressing
- ☐ Nut butter sandwiches
- ☐ Smoothies
- ☐ Baked goods, instead of eggs (1 tbsp. flax seed + 3 tbsp. water = 1 egg)

Other suggestions?

Ginger

Ginger has strong anti-inflammatory properties. Ginger is known to relieve nausea and digestive issues. Buy fresh ginger root or the powdered form. I buy fresh minced ginger sold in small jars.

Suggestions for Adding Ginger

- ☐ Hot or cold tea
- ☐ Salad dressing
- ☐ Sauces (especially Asian dishes)
- ☐ Stir fry
- ☐ Pumpkin pie spice—combination of cinnamon, ginger, nutmeg, and cloves

Other suggestions?

Herbs

Herbs add flavor and nutrition to foods. Herbs are leaves of plants. They possess anti-inflammatory and antioxidant elements as well as fiber. The most commonly used herbs include basil, cilantro, dill, fennel, marjoram, oregano, parsley, peppermint, rosemary, sage, tarragon, and thyme. All have health-promoting properties. Also, by adding herbs, you can reduce salt without forfeiting taste.

Dried herbs tend to be as beneficial as fresh. Since dried herbs have more concentrated flavors than fresh, use less when cooking.

Suggestions for Adding Herbs

- ☐ Sauces, soups, and stews
- ☐ Grain dishes
- ☐ Sandwich, burger, or wrap
- ☐ Seasoning on a salad or as "leafy greens" in the salad
- ☐ Salad dressings
- ☐ Boiled, baked, or mashed potatoes

- ☐ Vegetables before roasting or grilling
- ☐ Jarred pasta sauces or salsa
- ☐ Homemade nut-based or bean-based spreads and dips
- ☐ Iced or hot tea, or water
- ☐ Fresh fruit (see Summer Watermelon Salad on page 88)

Other suggestions?

Mushrooms

Mushrooms have unique anticancer properties. They contain antioxidants, the anti-inflammatory mineral selenium, and vitamin D. There are many varieties of mushrooms. Cremini, enoki, maitake, oyster, portobello, shiitake, and white button mushrooms are among the types most commonly eaten.

Suggestions for Adding Mushrooms

- ☐ Sauté with onions, garlic, and greens
- ☐ Mushroom burgers
- ☐ Grain dishes
- ☐ Sauces and one-pot meals
- ☐ Appetizers (see Stuffed Mushrooms on page 87)

Other suggestions?

Teas

Teas **have high nutritional profiles.** Green tea is the one often lauded, but oolong, white, and black teas are also beneficial. For optimal effectiveness, Dr. Servan-Schreiber recommends steeping green tea 5-10 minutes and drinking within an hour.[27] You can cold-brew tea in the refrigerator. Also, try adding loose tea leaves to food.

Suggestions for Adding Tea Leaves

☐ Smoothies

☐ Salad dressings

☐ Cooked grains

☐ Sauces

☐ Fresh fruit

☐ Baked goods

Other suggestions?

Tumeric

Turmeric has gained attention for its anti-inflammatory properties. In research studies, high doses of turmeric have reduced cancerous tumors. Curcumin is the active ingredient that makes turmeric so healthy. Buy turmeric root fresh or in powdered form. Powdered is more concentrated and stronger tasting. To enhance the absorption of turmeric:

·   add black pepper and

·   eat with a source of plant-based fat, such as with avocado, whole olives, walnuts, or seeds.

Note: Turmeric is significantly more effective when eaten, as opposed to ingested in supplement form.

Suggestions for Adding Turmeric

☐ Curry powder contains turmeric and other beneficial spices: cumin, coriander, red pepper, cardamom, ginger, cloves, nutmeg, cinnamon, and black pepper. Add to sauces, rice, grains, and soups.

☐ Stir-fry

☐ Baked potatoes

☐ Salad dressings (see No-Oil Balsamic Vinaigrette Dressing on page 90)

Other suggestions?

Colors

Eating foods with a range of colors provides you with a range of phytonutrients. Be aware of how your meal looks. If everything on your plate is one color, add food of another color. And don't be constrained by recipes. It's okay to add or substitute ingredients to compose a phytonutrient-hearty dish.

Suggestions for Adding Color

☐ Have a list of color-coded fruits and vegetables. "The Nutrition Rainbow" is available online through PCRM's *Cancer Project* [pcrm.org].

☐ Smoothies—multicolored fruits, plus mild-flavored leafy greens, pumpkin puree, or carrots.

☐ Chop or shred a variety of vegetables—onions, mushrooms, carrots, broccoli, cabbage, zucchini, peppers, tomatoes. Have them handy to add to cooked dishes, sandwiches, and cold salads.

☐ Add extra vegetables and herbs to jarred sauces and canned soup. I add extra tomatoes, corn, peppers, beans, and cilantro to jarred salsa.

☐ Put frozen vegetables and fruits in small glass containers in the refrigerator. Make them visible. I buy extra-large bags of frozen mixed berries and mixed vegetables. I refrigerate some in small glass containers. When family members see them, they eat them.

Other suggestions?

TRY-IT-OUT ACTIVITY

After reading the lists of suggestions:

1. For each food category, place a check next to one suggestion you'll try in the next week or two. Afterward, note whether you'll repeat it. Then, try another suggestion.

2. At the bottom of each list is space to add suggestions. *How can you introduce these foods into your day-to-day eating?* Use your imagination and then try your ideas.

Health Issues
Underweight

Do you have loss of appetite? Are you concerned about keeping sufficient weight on your body? If so, include these:

√ Plant foods with higher fat content—avocados, whole olives, nuts and seeds, nut butters, dried fruits.

√ Tofu—about half its calories are from fat.

√ Higher-fat milks—soy, almond, cashew—and yogurts.

√ Complex carbohydrates with concentrated calories— pasta, breads, crackers, cereals, baked goods.

√ Smoothies and juices (drink your calories).

√ Eat more often throughout the day.

Digestion

The most common complaint from people starting plant-based eating is the impact of fiber. Too much fiber can result in digestive stress—abdominal cramps, bloating, or diarrhea. Below are some guidelines to help you avoid distress:

√ Add fiber slowly to your diet.

√ Drink water throughout the day.

√ Be mindful if a particular food causes distress. If so, cut back or eliminate it until your body adjusts.

√ Soak dry beans in water before cooking. This helps reduce gassiness.

√ Chew your food slowly and thoroughly. This prevents swallowing excess air.

√ Choose foods that have less fiber and are easier to digest—white rice, refined flours, mashed potatoes, cooked vegetables, creamy soups, and smoothies.

√ Expect multiple bowel movements in a day. Remember, you are ridding your body of unwanted toxins.

√ Think of flatulence as a healthy by-product of fiber!

Also, you might have health issues that limit what you can eat. You could be on a soft-food diet following surgery. Or you might have scar tissue that compromises digestion. (That's me!) And you might be on a "low-residue" diet. A high-speed blender is invaluable in these situations. You retain vital nutrients while easing the load on your digestive tract. Blend any of the foods described in this chapter. Create smoothies, soups, sauces for cooked potatoes or rice, and nut butters. For easier digestion, grind oatmeal and cereals before cooking. Also, you still can eat those valuable greens. Grind them first before putting in a cold or hot dish.

Smoothies and Juicing

Generally, it is recommended that you eat your calories as opposed to drinking calories. Chewing food benefits digestion and absorption of nutrients. However, some people rely on a hearty and filling smoothie for breakfast each day. I enjoy smoothies as a refreshing and sweet-tasting treat.

Smoothies and juices have concentrated calories. They are helpful if you need to gain weight. Also, they are easily digested and beneficial for a compromised digestive system. My smoothie recipe is on page 94.

As the following chart illustrates, smoothies are superior to juices. Smoothies retain fiber and key nutrients. Plus, smoothies provide a greater feeling of fullness.

Smoothies	Juices
Fiber retained	Fiber removed
High natural sugars	Higher natural sugars
Fast way to get nutrients into bloodstream	Fastest way to get nutrients into bloodstream
Retains phytonutrients (in peel, seeds, stems)	Removes phytonutrients
Higher satiation (i.e., feeling of fullness)	Little satiation
Equipment: high-powered blender	Equipment: juicer

8

Work, Travel, and Dining Out

"Realize that every bite either enhances your health or sabotages it."
—Nedra H., plant-based eater

The world of work, travel, and social events is where your doggedness and determination come into play. Does it take effort and time? Yes. But your health is worth it!

Work and Travel: Plan Ahead

Prepare in advance. This is crucial for maintaining plant-based eating. You might not be accustomed to planning what to eat. If so, now is the time to develop new habits. Focus on creating a daily routine that is practical and realistic for you.

Always Have Food with You

Have two categories of food available: shelf-stable and fresh or frozen.

Shelf-stable items for your car, purse, coat pocket, briefcase, computer bag, travel bag, or desk at work. I stock these items:

- ☐ Small packages of nuts and dried fruit.

- ☐ Packaged snack bars without added fats and sugars. These are not easy to find. I buy Lara bars made from dried fruit, nuts, and spices. They are naturally sweetened and come in a variety of flavors. Also, look for healthier snack foods in the baby food aisles. The adults in my household are hooked on vanilla teething biscuits! They are organic, low fat, and with slight molasses sweetening.

☐ V8 juice (low-sodium) or other low-sodium, tomato-based juice in cans. Drink them when traveling. Also, use as a base for a quick soup.

☐ Pureed fruits and vegetables. Look in the baby aisle of the grocery store or online shopping site. You'll find combinations of pureed sweet potatoes, peas, spinach, pears, apples, kale, and more. Add to morning oatmeal, as a spread on bread, as a thickener for a quick soup, or over packaged rice or another grain.

☐ Single-serving applesauce or fruit chunks, without added sugar.

☐ Nondairy milk in shelf-stable packaging (soy, almond, rice, hemp, oat, and so on).

☐ Tea bags—green, oolong, or white.

☐ Soups—canned or shelf-stable packaging. The main problem is high sodium. Dilute saltiness by adding extra water and more vegetables. Or use a few spoonfuls of soup as a flavoring on top of potatoes, rice, or another grain. I recommend Dr. McDougall's packaged soups [www.shop.rightfoods.com].

☐ Precooked, packaged brown rice, quinoa, or other grain. For a quick meal, heat (or eat cold). Add canned vegetables, fruit, sauces, or flavorings.

Tip for leftover rice: In a microwaveable dish, combine rice, cinnamon, nuts, and dried fruit. Pour nondairy milk to soak. Refrigerate overnight. The next day, heat for a delicious rice pudding.

☐ Packages of unsweetened oatmeal. Or, better yet, fill a large zip-lock bag with oatmeal from home. (It's cheaper than the small packets of oatmeal.) Add cinnamon, nutritional yeast, ground flax seed, or other flavoring to the oatmeal bag. In your office or hotel room, put ½ cup of oatmeal in an empty cup, add water, and cook in microwave. If there is no microwave, heat water in a coffee maker.

☐ Favorite spices and flavorings. I travel with small containers of salsa, curry powder, and cinnamon.

☐ Dark chocolates, at least 70% cacao. Look for smaller, individually wrapped pieces.

Fresh or frozen food for meals and snacks for the upcoming day.

☐ Leftover meals from your freezer. Or keep several prepared entrees in the freezer at work. *PlantPure Nation* sells moderately priced plant-based meals. Have them shipped to your house or office.

☐ Fresh fruit that travels easily: apples, mandarin oranges, grapes, pears, plums, etc. I always have bananas for overnight trips. Though not the most nutritious fruit, bananas are easy to carry, filling, and versatile. I put slices on nut butter sandwiches or add to morning oatmeal.

☐ Fresh vegetables, such as miniature carrots, grape tomatoes, and sweet bell peppers.

☐ Individual portions of hummus, guacamole, and peanut butter.

☐ Slices of whole-grain bread or multigrain rolls or bagels. Store in a sandwich-sized bag. When hungry, eat plain or make a sandwich with salad ingredients.

☐ Potatoes provide satiation with nutrition. And they are versatile and easy to cook. In a hotel room or office, wrap a potato in a thick, absorbent hand towel. Microwave for several minutes. Let cool slightly, then unwrap and enjoy! I like spicy brown mustard on warm potatoes. Or eat with ketchup, salsa, salad dressing, curry powder, or other flavorings. Also, pop a wrapped baked potato in your bag or coat pocket for later.

Sweet potatoes vs. yams: Both are tuber root plants. The yam rarely is eaten outside of its native Africa. Sweet potatoes come in a variety of colors (purple, yellow, orange) and are packed with nutrients.

Use a small refrigerator and microwave. If your workplace does not have them, it's worthwhile to buy a small portable refrigerator and microwave. Search for advertised sales of dorm-sized refrigerators in late summer before colleges begin. Also, look for used refrigerators and microwaves at the end of a school year, when graduating students are cleaning out apartments. In a hotel, ask for a room refrigerator. Or, better yet, stay at suite or efficiency lodgings with kitchen amenities.

Prepare Meals Ahead of Time

Breakfast

Make it the night before, to eat hot or cold in the morning.

√   On multigrain bread, bagel, or wrap, put nut butter or another spread, no-sugar jam, and sliced fruit. Store in foil to reheat the next morning, or eat cold.

√   Oatmeal or other breakfast cereal.

Sally's Oatmeal Regimen: Starting Sunday evening, prepare bowls of oatmeal for three mornings (after three days, oatmeal gets too soggy). In small glass bowls with lids, combine ½ c. oatmeal, ½ c. water, ½ ripe banana, and a handful of frozen berries. Sprinkle pumpkin pie spice, ground flax seed, and nutritional yeast. In the morning, cook in the microwave for 1½ minutes. Add leafy greens if desired.

Oatmeal for Travel: In a coffee mug or Mason jar, combine ½ c. oatmeal, ½ c. nondairy milk, cinnamon, ground flax seed, chopped apples, raisins, and walnuts (or other fruits/nuts). Refrigerate overnight; eat cold or warm.

Lunch or Dinner

Pack food the night before. In the morning rush, you are less likely to prepare food for the day. Also, keep food in your office refrigerator and shelves. You want easy access to healthy, plant-based foods.

I packed the following foods for a workday (photo page 36). It's a lot of food! My motto is it's better to have an abundance of food at the ready. When hunger strikes, I want to eat something. And that "something" should satisfy both my appetite and my taste buds.

- √ Car ride to work: oatmeal/banana/berry bars (from my freezer)
- √ Morning snack: apple + half of the sandwich (tomato and cilantro/bean spread) + green tea
- √ Lunch: salad of lettuce, tomatoes, leftover potatoes, and vinaigrette dressing; fresh melon and blueberries
- √ Afternoon snack: the other half of sandwich
- √ Car ride home: apple

REFLECTION ACTIVITY

Which suggestions are the most helpful for you? Write down two specific actions you will do to prepare for upcoming work and travel.

1.

2.

As you develop routines for work and travel, share what you are doing on *PlantBasedEatingHub.com*.

Dining Out

You have less control of ingredients and cooking methods outside of your home. However, there are ways you can plan and make wise choices. Here are suggestions for how to maintain plant-centered eating when dining out.

Sit-Down Restaurants

Side dishes. Order from side dishes on the menu. You'll likely find potatoes, rice, beans, and various vegetables. Plus, your bill will be significantly lower than those of your seafood- and meat-eating companions.

Veggie burgers. Most chain restaurants have veggie burgers. Order without cheese or dairy-based sauce. Do pile on lettuce, tomatoes, pickles, and other vegetables.

Ethnic restaurants. Try Chinese, Indian, Italian, Thai, and similar restaurants. For Asian cuisine, choose tofu and vegetable options. For Italian cuisine, choose pasta with marinara sauce and a salad.

Call ahead. Find out if the restaurant caters to vegans. (The public understands "vegan" more than "plant-based.")

Server recommendations. Let your server know you are a vegan. Ask for their recommendation. Be aware that many vegan dishes are loaded with oil, salt, and sugar.

Special requests. Restaurants want to accommodate their customers (if they don't, avoid going there!). Ask the cook not to add oil and to sauté with water. Also, request substitutions, such as beans instead of cheese on your salad.

Chef's creation. Many chefs look forward to a creative challenge, especially at more upscale restaurants. Tell the server your diet restrictions. See if the chef will create a meal. I've had some delicious meals doing this. Often dining companions eye my plate and remark how tasty it looks!

Investigate. Check out menus and reviews online. Look at websites listing vegan restaurants. *Happycow.net* has international vegan restaurant listings.

Fast Food Restaurants

Pizza shops: Request pizza without cheese, but with lots of vegetables. (Yes, employees will look at you oddly!)

Sandwich or submarine shops: Order whole-grain bread with vegetables and sauces or condiments of your choice.

Coffee or doughnut shops: Many have oatmeal, whole-grain bagels, and fresh fruit. Some chains, such as Starbucks, carry prepackaged salads (use dressing sparingly) and vegetables with hummus.

Burger chains: Some have oatmeal. Most have types of salad (forgo meat and cheese). Burger King serves veggie burgers. Wendy's is my favorite because of plain baked potatoes.

Mexican restaurants: Bean burritos or rice bowls, with no added cheese.

Pita shops: Pitas with falafel or hummus.

Other options?

TRY-IT-OUT ACTIVITY

Sit-down restaurants: *Which of the eight suggestions have you done?* Try a new tactic the next time you dine out.

Fast food restaurants: *Do you know of other options?* If yes, share them on *PlantBasedEatingHub.com*.

Hospital Cafeterias

When I was writing this book, my husband had an unexpected hospital stay. I decided to add this section.

Hospitals are notorious for serving unhealthy food. If you are a patient, be persistent about requesting plant-centered meals. As a visitor, be creative in the cafeteria. Focus on salad ingredients, side dishes, breakfast cereal, soups, and prepackaged juices or smoothies.

Below are the meals I cobbled together during my husband's short stay. Also, I was glad I had travel food in my car for snacks.

Day 1

→ **Lunch:** navy bean soup + side order of rice + diced peppers, beets, spinach from the salad bar. I put rice and vegetables into the soup. This made for a heartier dish. Plus, it diluted excess saltiness.

→ **Snack:** oatmeal, with raisins and nuts from the salad bar (since it wasn't breakfast time, the cashier was reluctant to sell me oatmeal!).

→ **Dinner:** veggie burger on a soft bun (I asked the server for heartier bread) + salad bar (I added onions, tomatoes, and leafy lettuce to burger).

Day 2

→ **Breakfast:** oatmeal (I bought two packages, knowing that one wouldn't satisfy me) + bottled berry smoothie.

→ **Lunch:** vegetables in curry sauce over rice (I was lucky with this entree) + added chickpeas from salad bar.

Bottom line: ask for items, be inventive, and be determined. Your health is worth it.

9

Holidays, Celebrations, and Social Situations

"Eat by example. Lead by example."
—Sasha L., plant-based eater and cancer survivor

It's one thing to be committed to plant-based eating at home. It's another situation when you are attending holiday meals, celebrations, and other social situations.

Remember Roberta from chapter 2? Here are her comments about food, family, and friends:

> *Be steadfast with friends. Don't feel pressure to change back to your earlier way of eating. Be your own person. My family members get upset because of how I eat. Some won't even visit me (even though they have terrible health problems). I explain that I eat this way for my health and my life. For family get-togethers, I'll bring a huge salad with variety of vegetables. Of course, everyone eats it and enjoys it!*

You can have an active and satisfying social life while maintaining plant-based eating habits. Following are suggestions to help you:

Mantra Time!

The mantra you established in chapter 4 will come in handy during social situations. When you see luscious-looking desserts on a buffet table, remind yourself **why** you are committed to plant-based eating.

Tips for Social Situations

Don't arrive hungry. Eat something before socializing.

Before annual holiday meals, explain your new eating habits to family or friends. Why? So they won't expect you to eat the usual turkey, ham, deviled eggs, and so on. And tell them not to worry about accommodating you.

Bring a dish to share. (Something extra-tasty for people to ooh and aah about!)

Have your travel food ready. If there is nothing you want to eat, at least you'll have something to satisfy your hunger. I usually have multigrain bread along with a packet of raw nuts and raisins. Also, don't feel embarrassed. Explain that you have a new eating regimen—it's doctor's orders. (People don't argue with "doctor's orders.")

Remind yourself that your primary reason for being there is to enjoy the company of others. Food is secondary. As Nedra Hazlett says, "Don't let finding good food choices take the joy out of times with friends and family."

Responding to Negativity

Several years ago, I attended a December holiday party. The host is known for his cooking skills. A long-time friend offered me a plate of meat and cheese lasagna: "You *have to* taste Mike's lasagna. It's the best!" I declined politely. She then lifted a spoonful toward me: "just a bite won't hurt you." Again, I declined politely. (I did think: "a bite won't benefit me either.") My friend seemed dejected. I quickly changed the conversation.

Psychologist Doug Lisle[28] explains that food choices can represent status, even among the closest of friends and family. Some people might feel puzzled, irritated, and even excluded when they see you eating only healthful plant foods. What should you say or do when people make negative or guilt-laden remarks about your eating habits?

TRY-IT-OUT ACTIVITY

How would you react in these five situations? Write down what you would say or do. For comparison, my responses are at the end of this chapter. (Don't look until you've written yours!)

1. Host or hostess says: "I don't know what you eat. I don't know what to prepare for you." **Your response:**

2. Someone says: "You should enjoy yourself. Don't be so strict. Just take a bite." **Your response:**

3. Someone comments: "Here comes the picky eater!" **Your response:**

4. A person is quizzing you about your diet. He is challenging you about what is healthy eating. **Your response:**

5. Someone appears to be offended. You won't eat a dish she prepared "especially for you." **Your response:**

Sometimes people might seem snide or hostile toward your new lifestyle. When challenged, Doug Lisle recommends saying, "It seems to be working for me right now." This is a powerful response. You don't appear superior to the other person. And you are not insulting their food choices.

Others might ask you lots of questions. Some are curious and honestly interested. My experience is that most people's eyes glaze over when I describe plant-based eating. Saying, "I'll gladly explain it to you later" usually moves the conversation to another topic.

Be Committed

Moderate dietary changes lead to moderate health results. I want my chances of cancer recurrence to be as small as possible. Therefore, I choose to embrace a plant-based lifestyle fully. You decide how closely you want to follow a plant-based diet. Set your boundaries regarding what you will and will not consume. Nevertheless, know that sustained success is most likely to occur when you commit fully.[29]

There will be obstacles. Customs in society and among family and friends often work against maintaining this lifestyle. However, be committed. Own your identity as a plant-based eater. As with my example about the holiday lasagna, avoid eating foods just to please others. Don't let peoples' expectations weaken your dedication. It is your health and your choice. Embolden yourself. Take pride in your commitment to such a healthy and powerful way of eating.

SALLY'S RESPONSES

First, smile! It's not useful to be confrontational or defensive. Plus, social gatherings aren't an occasion to educate others and try to change minds.

1. **Don't worry about me.** Is it okay if I bring a dish to share with everyone? If you want to learn more about what I eat, I'll be glad to talk with you sometime.

2. **I am enjoying myself.** I am not depriving myself. I'm committed to plant-based eating because I feel so much better.

3. **I prefer to call myself a healthy eater.** I prefer foods that might be different from what you are accustomed to. I am choosy about what I eat, and I feel so much better! (Don't spend your time engaged in a no-win argument.)

4. **I've had cancer. This made me think differently about food.** It seems we are not going to agree, which is okay. If you want more information about plant-based eating, I'll gladly provide you resources from experts.

5. **I'm sorry, but I want to keep on track.** Your dish looks delicious. I'm sure other people will thoroughly enjoy it. A plant-based diet is doctor's orders! (You will not be lying. Plenty of knowledgeable physicians prescribe plant-based eating. Though it might not be **your** doctor!)

10

Stress and Comfort Foods

Pam switched to a plant-based diet two years ago. Since then, she's noticed striking changes in her mental well-being:

I'm amazed at the improvement in my mental energy. I'm sharper and more focused. Sometimes I do feel a little down, but I get over it quicker. My day-to-day moods have improved dramatically.

Like Pam, I've noticed my mental well-being has improved with plant-based eating.

There is abundant research linking food with moods and emotional health. Studies indicate that people eating diets high in processed foods, fried foods, sugar, and refined grains have a significant risk for depression and anxiety. On the flip side, people eating more fruit and vegetables have increased levels of happiness and satisfaction. What you eat can improve depression, anxiety, emotional well-being, and overall daily functioning.[30]

Does eating fewer healthy foods cause depression and anxiety? Or do depressed, anxious people crave unhealthy foods? Either way, it's to your advantage to choose healthier, plant-based foods, especially when feeling stressed or anxious.

Stress and Food Choices

There is a reason we crave processed foods high in fat, sugar, and salt. The taste provides us with immediate pleasure. But the blissful flavors of sugar, fat, and salt are short-lived. We then are left with uneven blood sugar levels, lack of energy, and unhappiness with ourselves. These negative physical and mental feelings often result in consuming *more* comfort foods.[31]

1. **Reason** → feeling stressed, angry, fearful, or anxious

2. **Action** → eating comfort foods (highly processed, high sugar, fat, and salt)

3. **Immediate effect** → feelings of pleasure and better mood (though short-term!)

4. **Continued effect** → uneven blood sugar, feelings of sluggishness, foggy brain, and self-loathing. This leads back to feeling stressed, anxious, craving comfort foods, and so on.

TRY-IT-OUT ACTIVITY

1. The left column of the following chart lists foods that people commonly crave. *Which ones do you crave?* In the right column, *which of the alternative foods appeal to you?* Also, jot down more ideas for healthier substitutes.

2. *When you eat healthier comfort foods, do you notice a difference in your mood?* If so, what's the difference?

Food Cravings and Healthier Alternatives

Craving	Healthier Alternative
Chocolate	Dark chocolate (at least 70% cacao), small amounts Unsweetened cocoa in nondairy milk, cold or hot Cacao and date cookies and brownies (page 93)
Refined sugar	Naturally sweet fruits (pineapple, berries, watermelon) Naturally sweet vegetables (carrots, corn Carbonated water sweetened with mint leaves or splashes of fruit juices Dried fruit
Refined baked goods (cake, cookies, pastries)	Fiber-rich carbohydrates such as oatmeal, sweet potatoes, or multigrain pasta Baked goods sweetened with dates, ripe bananas, or applesauce (page 93) Whole-grain baked goods
Cheese	Nondairy or vegan cheeses (page 92) Hummus (has a cheese-like consistency when warmed)
Creamy foods	Creamed soups and sauces from cauliflower, potatoes, avocados, or nondairy milk Vegan-style macaroni and cheese Puddings from nondairy milk
Ice cream and frozen treats	Sorbet or smoothies from frozen bananas and berries (page 94) Frozen grapes Frozen bananas rolled in cocoa or coconut Frozen cacao, date, and nut bars (page 93)
Caffeine	Lower-caffeinated teas Decaffeinated coffee Sparkling water with a splash of fruit juice or pieces of whole fruit
Salt	Pretzels or crackers that are salt-free or have lower salt content Popcorn—either air-popped or popped in a paper bag in a microwave. Sprinkle with cinnamon, nutritional yeast, smoky paprika, pumpkin pie spice, or other flavoring
Any others?	

Be aware of your moods, emotions, and food cravings. Next time you feel stressed, notice which foods you automatically reach for. Stop and consider whether you want to substitute something else. Stock up on foods that are healthy, yet pleasurable to eat. (My go-to comfort food is oatmeal cooked with bananas, berries, and nondairy milk. To me, it's sweet, creamy, and satisfying.)

Develop a pattern that strengthens your physical and emotional health:

1. **Reason** → feeling stressed, angry, fearful, or anxious
2. **Action** → eating healthy comfort foods (minimally processed; low sugar, fat, and salt)
3. **Effect** → stable blood sugar; more energy, alertness, and self-satisfaction

Finally, be kind to yourself. Be committed to eating healthily, yet allow yourself to be imperfect. I often hear people remark, "I've been bad" or "I've fallen off the wagon." There is no wagon to fall off on this journey. Remember: you are traveling on your individual path toward health and well-being.

11

Find a Like-Minded Community

"Nothing compares to the camaraderie of like-minded people."
—Joe W., cancer survivor and plant-based eater

Remember Marty from chapter two? She is the colon cancer survivor who never felt better after embracing a plant-based lifestyle. She is part of my plant-based support group. Here is the rest of her story:

However, I got cocky! I treated myself to seafood during a beach vacation. And then began eating more and more processed foods, especially lots of cheese. My work changed, adding more stress. I ate fast food again. I was gaining weight back and feeling poorly. When I found out my blood pressure had zoomed upward, I did some honest soul searching. I knew I had to get back to plant-based eating. I felt better within weeks. Currently, I've lost 50 pounds and my blood pressure is normal. And I'm confident that I won't lapse again. I'm committed to making plant-based eating work for me and members of my household. My advice to others:

- *Find much-needed support. Look for face-to-face and online communities.*
- *Set your boundaries. Decide what you will and won't eat. Let others know. Sometimes you need to be assertive.*

Approximately 2% of adults are vegetarian or vegan. Personal health is the main reason they choose meatless diets. On the other hand, 10% of adults are **former** vegetarians or vegans. Why did they revert to eating meat again? Primarily because they felt isolated and weren't involved with people of similar lifestyle. In addition, nearly all former vegetarians/vegans want to return to meatless eating.[32]

Don't be a **former** plant-based eater. Do seek out others who follow a similar way of eating. Just as your food desires change, so will your social desires. You probably will want to be among like-minded people. Interacting with other plant-based eaters is a great motivational tool. Share meals and recipes, offer advice, and support one another. You'll develop a strong sense of camaraderie. Being part of a plant-based community can be key to sustaining your healthy lifestyle. In other words, find your tribe!

How to Find Your Community

Here are six suggestions to get you started:

Find local meet-ups. Search for local events on meetup.com. Vegan meet-ups are widespread. Also, search for whole food nutrition, plant-based nutrition, raw food, or similarly named groups. It can be intimidating to attend a new event. Know that people are eager to meet others and find common ground. Health-conscious people tend to be accepting and friendly. I've met many wonderful people at meet-up events nearby, as well as when traveling.

Find plant-based eating classes and workshops. Explore local adult education classes, community library presentations, and educational events at health-care centers. See if there are Physician Committee for Responsible Medicine's "Food for Life" classes near you. These classes cover useful information about foods and health, cooking demonstrations, and recipes. They currently are offered in Australia, Canada, the United Kingdom, and the United States. (pcrm.org)

Attend educational conferences. See the listing in chapter 12. Also, go to vegan festivals. Be aware people have differing priorities at vegan events. Some are concerned primarily about animals, others about health, and still others about the environment.

Find online communities. Check out the *PlantPure Communities Pod Program* [plantpurepods.com]. This is a collaborative network offering guidance and support. There might be a local "pod" near you. Also, search for whole food, plant-based groups on Facebook.

Visit vegan-friendly restaurants. Meet local like-minded eaters. When traveling, patronize vegan restaurants and retail establishments. Chapter 12 has a list of online travel guides.

Create a support group. Ask friends, colleagues, or family members if they want to join. Most people are concerned about eating healthily. Being part of a supportive, cohesive group is appealing to many. Steps for organizing a plant-based group include:

- Find a gathering space (library, community building, church, supermarket, or home).
- Set a regular day and time to meet.
- Give people a reason to attend (i.e., topics for discussion or potluck meals).
- Publicize via Facebook, meet-up sites, flyers, e-invites, and word-of-mouth.
- Request that everyone share experiences and bring a friend.

TRY-IT-OUT ACTIVITY

Which of the six suggestions are practical and realistic for you? Put a check next to those you are ready to do. Then, go ahead and try it out!

Also, as you adopt plant-based eating habits, you'll influence family and friends over time. For instance, I recently invited friends to a last-minute summer potluck dinner at my house. None are purely plant-based eaters. Everyone brought a dish to share. We ended up with a beautiful array of delicious and filling plant-based dishes. One person did bring meat, but I noticed that only he ate it. A friend commented afterward that because of my influence, friends now eat ever more nutritious—and flavorful—foods. This brought a smile to my face!

Sustaining Your Plant-Based Eating

What motivates you to continue your plant-based journey? Here are answers from members of my plant-based community:

- "My husband and I reinforce each other. We try to be role models for our family." (Linda A.)

- "My sister died from cancer. I know that eating plants helps prevent disease." (Donna P.)

- "Eating this way is my food and my medicine." (Roberta W.)

- "I loved meat, but it tried to kill me! Great bloodwork motivates me." (Nedra H.)

- "I want to live longer to see my grandchildren grow up." (Lulu H.)

- "Attending this support group." (Donna W.)

REFLECTION ACTIVITY

Refer to chapter 4 activities, when you were starting your plant-based journey.

1. On page 22, you considered the importance of food in your lifestyle. Review your answers. *At this point, do you notice changes regarding your view of food?* If so, add your comments.

2. On page 23, you identified what motivates you to change eating habits. If now you have other reasons, add them to your list.

Closing Thoughts

Here's a summary of what I've learned during my plant-based journey:

→ Foods consumed day-to-day have an immediate and lasting impact on your health and well-being.

→ Food choices affect physical, mental, and emotional health. All three are intertwined.

→ What you **do** eat (whole grains, legumes, vegetables, fruits) is as important as what you **don't** eat (highly processed, high fat, high sugar, low fiber).

→ Plant foods can prevent and even reverse disease.

→ Plant-based eating changes taste buds and food desires.

→ Plant-based eating can be simple and inexpensive.

→ Food choices have a powerful impact. I now think of food as tasty, nourishing, multicolored medicine for my body.

→ To maintain healthy eating habits, seek out supportive, health-conscious people.

What have you learned?

What has been significant for you? Share your knowledge with family and friends. Let them know what you've accomplished. Plus, post your thoughts and questions on *PlantBasedEatingHub.com*.

12

Use These Resources

Matthew, a cancer survivor, offered these words:

I was going through treatment for cancer five years ago. It was a scary time for me. A friend told me about the film Forks Over Knives. *I watched it and was astounded. The film shows how a whole food plant-based diet can reverse chronic illnesses. I then read* The China Study. *I didn't need any more convincing. I've been a plant-based eater ever since. I enjoy the many free and helpful online resources: newsletters, videos, and recipe collections.*

As you move along in your journey, I encourage you to make use of experts and advocates in the field of plant-based nutrition. This chapter contains listings of select resources. There are many more. As the practice of plant-based eating spreads, so do related cookbooks, blogs, and organizations.

REFLECTION ACTIVITY

Return to page 8. Review what you wrote for the question: **What is a burning question you have at this point?**

Can you answer this question now? If not, see if you find the answer using these resources.

Organizations

Forks Over Knives: The 2011 documentary highlights health benefits of plant-based diets in overcoming the epidemic of chronic, degenerative diseases—including cancer. The film is enlightening and enjoyable. The website contains articles, recipes, and information about educational programs. *Forks Over Knives: The Cookbook* (2012) is comprehensive and useful. (My go-to cookbook!)

John McDougall, MD: McDougall's website includes a free 10-day meal plan, articles, recipes, information about residential programs at Dr. McDougall's Health and Medical Center, and webinars. Along with Mary McDougall, he is author of *The Starch Solution* (2012) and *The Healthiest Diet on the Planet* (2016).

North American Vegetarian Society (NAVS): The annual Summerfest conference includes an array of informative speakers from experts in the field of plant-based eating.

NutritionFacts.org: Michael Greger, MD, analyzes and summarizes the latest research in daily videos and blogs that are factual, consumer friendly, and without commercial bias. This is my go-to site for evidence-based information on a wide range of nutrition-related topics. I recommend his comprehensive book, *How Not to Die: Discover the Foods Scientifically Proven to Prevent and Reverse Disease* (2015).

Physicians Committee for Responsible Medicine (PCRM): Nutrition research and healthful eating advocacy founded by Neal Barnard, MD. The 21-Day Vegan Kickstart provides free meal plans, recipes, tips, and support. The Cancer Project is a valuable resource. Look for "Food for Life" classes near you. Barnard Medical Center, located in Washington, DC, offers medical care with prevention and nutrition in mind.

PlantPure Nation: A 2015 documentary and movement to promote the power of plant-based eating to repair our health-care crisis. The website includes a 21-Day Jumpstart Challenge as well as meal-starter kits and recipes. Their frozen entrees are moderately priced and very convenient.

Kim Campbell's *PlantPure Nation Cookbook* (2015) and *PlantPure Kitchen Cookbook* (2017) contain practical, easy-to-follow recipes. The PlantPure Communities Pod Program is a network of groups and people offering guidance and support for one another.

Plantrician Project: Contains abundant plant-based nutrition resources.

T. Colin Campbell Center for Nutrition Studies: Based on Campbell's groundbreaking research, the organization promotes optimal nutrition via science-based education, advocacy, and research. You'll find recipes, articles, and the eCornell Plant-Based Nutrition Certificate.

Books and Magazines

Anticancer: A New Way of Life by David Servan-Schreiber, MD, PhD, Penguin Group, 2008.

The Blue Zones: 9 Lessons for Living Longer from the People Who've Lived the Longest by Dan Buettner, National Geographic Society, 2012.

The Cheese Trap: How Breaking a Surprising Addiction Will Help You Lose Weight, Gain Energy, and Get Healthy by Neal Barnard, MD, Grand Central Life & Style, 2017.

The China Study: Startling Implications for Diet, Weight Loss and Long-Term Health by T. Colin Campbell, PhD, and Thomas Campbell, Ben Bella Books, 2006.

Dr. Neal Barnard's Program for Reversing Diabetes: The Scientifically Proven System for Reversing Diabetes without Drugs by Neal Barnard, MD, Rodale Books, 2007.

Naked Food magazine by Margarita Restrepo is a digital and print publication for whole foods, plant-based lifestyle. [nakedfoodmagazine.com]

Prevent and Reverse Heart Disease: The Revolutionary, Scientifically Proven, Nutrition-Based Cure by Caldwell B. Esselstyn, Jr, MD, Avery, 2007.

Whole: Rethinking the Science of Nutrition by T. Colin Campbell, PhD, and Howard Jacobson, PhD, BenBella Books, 2013.

Cookbooks, Recipes, and Meal Plans

Appetite for Reduction: 125 Fast and Filling Low-Fat Vegan Recipes by Isa Chandra, Da Capo Press, 2011.

Cancer Survivors Guide: Foods That Help You Fight Back by Neal Barnard, MD, and Jennifer Reilly, Book Publishing Co., 2008.

The China Study Cookbook: Over 120 Whole Food, Plant-Based Recipes by LeAnne Campbell, Ben Bella Books, 2013.

The China Study Quick and Easy Cookbook: Cook Once, Eat All Week with Whole Food, Plant-Based Recipes by Del Sroufe, Ben Bella Books, 2015.

Crazy Sexy Wellness Revolution by Kris Carr. A late-stage cancer survivor, Carr posts blogs, videos, and recipes about wellness and plant-based living. [kriscarr.com]

e-Book: *Whole Food, Plant Based on $5 a Day* by Emma Rouche. [plantplate.com]

Forks Over Knives has an online meal planner, with options for individuals, couples, or families. You can indicate an intolerance for nuts, soy, or gluten. The recipe app is easy to use, with new recipes added regularly.

Get Healthy, Go Vegan Cookbook: 125 Easy and Delicious Recipes to Jump-Start Weight Loss and Help You Feel Great by Neal Barnard, MD and Robyn Webb, Da Capo Press, 2010.

Happy Herbivore: Lindsay Nixon simplifies meal planning with her "Meal Mentor" plans, easy recipes, and practical information. I recommend her cookbook series (Ben Bella Books). She advocates pursuing "progress, not perfection!"

Oh She Glows by Angela Liddon. Most of Liddon's online recipes also are free of gluten, soy, and processed foods.

Protective Diet: The Oil-, Sugar- and Nut-Free Plant-Based Plan by Julie Marie Christensen.

Online Shopping

Amazon: You can find almost anything in the world's largest marketplace. Be aware of added shipping costs. And some products are priced significantly higher than what stores charge.

Thrive Marketplace: Specializes in natural and organic food and specialty items at reduced prices. There is a yearly membership fee.

Vitacost: Carries food items, though specializes in supplements.

Online Cooking Courses

Culinary Rx [plantrician.rouxbe.com]

Forks Over Knives Plant-Based Cooking Course [forksoverknives.com/cooking-course]

Online Educational Summits

Food Revolution Summit, hosted by John and Ocean Robbins [foodrevolutionsummit.org]

Lifestyle Medicine Summit, hosted by Lifestyle Prescriptions Foundation [lifestyleprescriptions.org/summit]

Plant-Based Transformation Summit, hosted by Margot Freitag [taigawholehealth.com/plantbasedtransformation]

Online Travel Guides

Happy Cow: listing of vegan dining options worldwide.

PCRM's 2014 Airport Travel Guide lists healthy eating options at 23 busy airports.

Vegan Travel: reviews about global dining, lodging, and events.

TripAdvisor: search for vegan restaurants and travel information.

For Health-Care Professionals

Conferences and organizations where physicians, nurses, and health-care providers can learn about plant-based eating. Most offer continuing education units. Share this list with your health-care practitioners.

American College of Lifestyle Medicine [lifestylemedicine.org]

Angiogenesis Foundation: "Conquering cancer by starving the blood vessels that feed tumor growth." [angio.org]

Dr. McDougall's Health and Medical Center Professionals Weekend [drmcdougall.com]

International Plant-Based Nutrition Healthcare Conference [pbnhc.com]

Nutrition and Health Conference [nutritionandhealthcof.org]

Physicians Committee for Responsible Medicine, Physician Resources + International Conference on Nutrition in Medicine [pcrm.org/for_physicians]

Plant-Based Prevention of Disease Conference [preventionofdisease.org]

Vegetarian Nutrition Dietetic Practice Group of the Academy of Nutrition and Dietetics [vegetariannutrition.net]

FINAL ACTIVITY: FIND A PLANT-BASED HEALTH-CARE PROVIDER

It's not easy to locate a health-care practitioner who understands and supports plant-based eating. Look up practitioners on **plantbaseddoctors.org**. *Are any near you?*

Sample Plant-Based Recipes

Breakfast

Banana Pancakes

4 ripe bananas, mashed
2¼ c water
¼ c unsweetened applesauce
2 tsp vanilla extract
2 c flour of choice (whole wheat, oat, chickpea, etc.)
1½ tbsp baking powder
2 tsp cinnamon

Combine wet ingredients in a bowl. Add dry ingredients; mix well. In non-stick pan, cook over low to medium heat, about 3 minutes each side. *(by Linda Jones)*

Tofu Scramble

1 14-oz block extra-firm tofu
1 small onion, chopped
1 small green bell pepper, chopped finely
1 small red bell pepper, chopped finely
1 small carrot, chopped
½ tsp ground coriander
½ tsp ground cumin
1½ tsp ground turmeric
1 tsp garlic powder
salt/pepper

Place tofu on a plate lined with several layers of paper towels (to absorb liquid). In pan, cook onion, peppers, and carrots until softened, 3-4 minutes. Stir in cumin; cook for 1 minute. Stir in crumbled tofu, then turmeric (gives egg-like color). Stir often, until heated, 1-2 minutes. Stir in garlic powder; season with salt/pepper. *(by Brittany Jaroudis @ thejaroudis.com)*

Lunch and Dinner

Very Quick Sweet Potato Bisque

> 1 14-oz can pureed sweet potatoes
> 14 oz of water, broth, or nondairy milk (for creamier soup)
> ½ tsp curry powder

In blender, empty sweet potatoes, curry powder, and liquid of choice. Blend until smooth. Add to taste: jarred salsa, diced tomatoes, and other frozen or fresh vegetables. Heat and eat! *(by Sally Lipsky)*

Chunky Veggie Soup

> 1 onion, chopped
> 3 garlic cloves, minced
> ½ inch fresh ginger, peeled/minced
> 1 tbsp cumin
> 1 tsp turmeric
> ½ tsp coriander
> salt/pepper to taste
> 3 large carrots, chopped
> 3 celery ribs, chopped
> ½ head red cabbage, cut in chunks
> 3-4 potatoes, diced
> 6 c vegetable broth

In large saucepan, sauté onions, garlic, and ginger in water or broth until partially cooked. Add cumin, turmeric, and coriander. Add salt/pepper. Add carrots, celery, and cabbage; sauté briefly. Add potatoes and broth. Bring to boil; simmer on low until vegetables are cooked (about 30 minutes). Adjust spices to taste. *(by Arlene Holtz)*

Curried Indian Potato Stew

2 28-oz cans no-salt chopped tomatoes
2 14-oz cans no-salt garbanzo beans
frozen cauliflower (1½ lb), peas (¼ lb), onions (¼ lb)
3-4 c cooked potatoes
salt-free curry spice mix

Microwave, steam, or boil potatoes; cut in 1-inch pieces. (Or cook diced potatoes in the pot with just enough water to cover.) When potatoes are done, put other ingredients in pot and heat. Add seasoning; top with fresh cilantro. *(with permission from Jeff Novick, MS, RDN, www.JeffNovick.com)*

Black Olive and Corn Stew

1 15-oz can chickpeas or other bean, drained/rinsed
1 15-oz can diced tomatoes, drained
1 15-oz can corn, drained
1 6-oz can black olives, drained
1 green pepper, cubed **or** 2 pieces roasted pepper from jar
1 tbsp tomato paste
1 tbsp dry onion flakes
1 tbsp dry garlic flakes
2 tbsp soy sauce
⅛ tsp red pepper flakes
1 tbsp sugar
1 tsp cumin
1 tbsp balsamic vinegar
salt/pepper to taste
1 tsp dry oregano (optional)

Combine all ingredients in sauté pan; cook until most of liquid evaporates and sauce thickens. For thinner sauce, heat until flavors blend; don't evaporate liquid. Serve over rice, quinoa, bread, or tortilla. *(by Lourdes Herold @ Lulu Cooks and Tells)*

Easy Pineapple Rice

Hollow out a whole pineapple; chop the inside fruit. Combine: cooked brown rice, black beans, chopped multi-colored peppers, pineapple, and mango. Stir in pineapple juice and a splash of teriyaki sauce, to taste. *(by Nedra Hazlett)*

Slow Cooker Rice and Beans

1 lb dry red kidney beans
1 red pepper, chopped
1 green pepper, chopped
1 small onion, chopped
3 cloves garlic, minced
3 stalks celery, chopped
1 tbsp Cajun seasoning
7 c water or vegetable broth

Combine ingredients in crockpot. Cover. Cook on high 7 hours until beans are tender. Serve with cooked brown rice and chopped kale greens. *(by Roberta Woodfork)*

Easy Salsa Tofu

1 package extra-firm tofu, cut in ½ inch cubes
1 c salsa

Combine tofu and salsa in non-stick frying pan. Cook over med-high heat, covered. Flip tofu after 15 minutes. Cook 10 minutes more, until edges are brown and crusty. Eat as a main dish; over potatoes, rice or other grain; or in a hot sandwich or wrap. *(by Kylie Lichtenstein)*

Stuffed Green Peppers

4 green peppers
¾ c mushrooms of choice
¼ c dates
1 shallot, chopped finely
1 clove garlic, chopped finely
1½ c tomato sauce
1½ c cooked brown or wild rice
salt/pepper to taste

Preheat oven to 350⁰F. Remove seeds, tops, and membranes from peppers. Parboil in water until tender, about 10 minutes. Sauté mushrooms, dates, shallot, garlic, and salt/pepper in pan. Use a little water, if needed. Mix with rice. For each pepper: fill halfway with rice/veggie mixture, add tomato sauce, fill to top with rice mixture, then add more sauce. Add remaining sauce to bottom of baking dish. Bake 20-25 minutes. *(by Roberta Woodfork)*

Stuffed Mushrooms

8 cremini or white button mushrooms
4 stalks green onions, chopped finely

Preheat oven to 375⁰F. Clean mushrooms; remove and chop stems. Combine: chopped stems, green onions, and Parmesan filling. Fill each mushroom cap with spoonful of the mixture. Bake 12-15 minutes.

Vegan Parmesan filling: 1 c walnuts, 1 tbsp nutritional yeast, + ¼ tsp garlic powder. In blender, mix until a coarse texture. *(by Lourdes Herold @ Lulu Cooks and Tells)*

"Polentil" Veggie Bake

Great for guests or a special occasion!

Red Lentil Sauce: Bring 1 c lentils and 4 c water to a boil in large pot. Cover, reduce heat, simmer 20-25 minutes until lentils are tender. Add:

> 1 large onion, chopped
> 1 red pepper, chopped finely
> 2-3 garlic cloves, minced
> 1 26-oz can chopped tomatoes
> 1 large carrot, grated
> 2 tsp Italian seasoning
> 1 small zucchini, grated
> 2 tbsp tomato paste

Bring to a boil, cover, reduce heat. Simmer for 1 hour, until thick.

Spinach/Mushroom Filling: 2 8-oz packages of mushrooms + 1 10-oz package frozen spinach. Simmer mushrooms in pan, with small amount of water, until soft. Cook frozen spinach according to package. Combine spinach and mushrooms, set aside.

Polenta Layers: Cook packaged polenta (such as Bob's Red Mill Polenta Corn Grits)—2 c polenta to 6 c water.

Assemble Casserole: Preheat oven to 350⁰F. In 9 x 13" pan, pour thin layer of red lentil sauce on bottom. Spoon half of polenta on top, flatten with spatula. Add spinach/mushroom filling. Top with lentil sauce. Add rest of polenta. Top with remaining lentil sauce. Bake 30 minutes. *(by Linda Askren)*

Summer Watermelon Salad

Cut up and combine: watermelon, tomatoes, mint, and basil. Sprinkle with lemon juice. *(by Nedra Hazlett)*

Quinoa Carrot Salad

1 c quinoa, cooked
1 cucumber, diced
1 c shredded carrot
1 c grape tomatoes **or** 1 c sun-dried tomatoes
fresh parsley
1 scallion, sliced
salt/pepper to taste
nutritional yeast

Roast grape tomatoes at 400°F. for 18 minutes *or* puree sun-dried tomatoes. In a bowl, combine quinoa, cucumber, carrot, tomato, parsley, and scallion. Add Citrus Salad Dressing (see next section) and salt/pepper. Top with nutritional yeast. *(by Donna Whiteside)*

Mediterranean Couscous Salad

1 c Israeli couscous
1 c each red + yellow bell pepper, diced
1 c broccoli florets, cut in small pieces
1 c canned artichoke hearts, diced large
½ c Kalamata olives, sliced
1 c grape tomatoes, halved
1 c kale, chopped (raw or steamed lightly)
½ avocado, diced
¼ c slivered almonds or sesame seeds (optional)

Cook couscous according to package. Combine vegetables (not tomatoes) with cooled couscous. Add Mediterranean Salad Dressing (see next section). Top with tomatoes. Sprinkle nuts/seeds. *(by Susan Greenberg)*

Dressings, Dips, and Spreads

Citrus Salad Dressing

Mix 2 tbsp lemon or orange juice + 3 tbsp vegetable broth. *(by Donna Whiteside)*

Mediterranean Salad Dressing

3 tbsp fresh lemon juice
2 tbsp water
2-3 cloves minced garlic
1 tsp dried oregano
1 tsp dried mint
salt/pepper to taste

Mix ingredients. *(by Susan Greenberg)*

No-Oil Balsamic Vinaigrette Dressing

1 c balsamic vinegar
⅓ c water
⅓-½ c Dijon mustard *(emulsifier)*
1 tbsp minced garlic *(allium family)*
½ tsp minced ginger *(antioxidant)*
½ tsp ground flax seed *(lignan, omega-3 fatty acids)*
½ tsp sesame seeds *(fat-soluble, aids absorption)*
½ tsp turmeric *(anti-inflammatory)*
black pepper *(aids absorption of turmeric)*
squirt lemon juice *(aids absorption of leafy greens)*
sun-dried tomatoes *(lycopene)*
herbs, fresh or dried *(more antioxidants!)*

Combine ingredients in jar. Shake and serve. Besides salads, I add to soups, one-pot meals, and grain dishes. *(by Sally Lipsky)*

Ranch Dressing

1 c raw cashews, soaked in water for 1 hour
¼ c water
2 tbsp lemon juice
½ tsp garlic powder
½ tsp onion powder
1 tbsp chopped fresh basil
1 tbsp chopped fresh dill
salt to taste

In food processor or blender, mix ingredients until smooth. Experiment with various seasonings, fresh or dried herbs, and whether to add more or less water. Use this as a spread on crackers or sandwiches, or a dip for fresh vegetables. *(with permission from Janet McKee, Fabulous Recipes for Vibrant Health, 2010)*

Mixed Berries Jalapeno Chia Spread

6 oz blackberries
8 oz strawberries
2 tbsp bottled jalapeno slices
juice of ½ lemon
6 tbsp maple syrup
2 tbsp chia seeds
salt to taste

Place ingredients in blender; pulse until fine. *(by Lourdes Herold @ Lulu Cooks and Tells)*

Creamy Cashew Nut Cheese

1 c raw cashew nuts
1 tbsp tahini
1 tbsp nutritional yeast
¼-½ c water
juice of 1 lime or lemon
salt/pepper to taste

In a food processor or blender, combine all ingredients until creamy. Adjust water for desired thickness and texture. *(with permission from Deliciously Ella @ deliciouslyella.com)*

Plant-Based Cream Cheese

1 cheesecloth
2 5-oz containers plain, plant-based yogurt

Open cheesecloth; place over a deep bowl. Scoop yogurt on top. Tie cheesecloth on a spoon sitting on the top. Yogurt drips into the bowl, making ¼-½ c liquid. Refrigerate 24 hours. Transfer thickened yogurt from cheesecloth to bowl. Spread on toasted bagel or bread; top with fruit. *(by Brittany Jaroudis @ thejaroudis.com)*

Easy Bean Dip

1 15-oz can cannelloni beans, drained/rinsed
1 15-oz can garbanzo beans, drained/rinsed
3 tbsp Dijon mustard
2 garlic cloves, minced
2 tsp fresh lemon juice
1 tsp ground dill
1 tsp paprika

Puree all ingredients in blender or food processor, until smooth. Serve with raw vegetables, baked corn chips or pretzels, or use as a spread on sandwiches or wraps. *(by Brittany Jaroudis @ thejaroudis.com)*

Desserts and Snacks

Raw Choco Bites

1 carrot
3 figs + 3 dates **or** 6 dates
1 banana
½ c rolled oats
2 tsp raw cacao
shredded coconut (optional)

Chop carrot in large pieces. In blender or food processor, mix carrots and dates/figs for 10-15 seconds, until minced. Set aside. In large bowl, add banana and oats; mash with fork or bare hands. Add carrot mixture and raw cacao. Blend until mixture is uniform. Shape into 1-inch round bites. Pour coconut (if using) in small bowl and roll each bite until covered. *(with permission from Naked Food Magazine, nakedfoodmagazine.com)*

Raw Chewy Chocolate Brownies

2 c raw walnuts
2 c dates, soaked in water to soften (pits removed)
1 c cocoa powder or raw cacao powder
1 tbsp vanilla extract
pinch salt

In blender or food processor, grind walnuts. Add drained dates and remaining ingredients. Blend. If more moisture needed, add small amount of water from dates. Press into 9 x 9" pan. Cut into 16 squares. For a cold treat, freeze. *(with permission from Janet McKee @ Sanaview.com)*

Nondairy Ice Cream

1½ frozen bananas
¼ c almond milk
flavoring: 3 frozen strawberries *or* 3 tsp cacao powder
      or 2 tsp vanilla extract

In high-speed blender, mix until smooth: frozen bananas, almond milk, and a flavoring. Freeze 15 minutes.

For banana split: Scoop three flavors of ice cream onto a banana, cut in half lengthwise. Add toppings of your choice (nuts, coconut, cherries). *(by Brittany Jaroudis @ thejaroudis.com)*

Sally's Smoothie

1 c baby carrots
1 ripe banana
1 tbsp dried green tea leaves (I empty a tea bag)
1 tbsp nutritional yeast
lemon or lime slice
⅓ c plant-based milk (modify for desired thickness)
1 c frozen mixed berries
scoop of ice cubes
optional: nut butter, leafy greens, apple chunks (or other
      fruit), mint leaves (or other herb), cacao powder

Starting with carrots, put ingredients in high-powered blender. Blend until smooth.

Banana Oat Bars

*I make a double batch, freezing bars in plastic
sandwich bags for a grab-and-go snack.*

1 c ground oats
1 c whole oats
2 ripe bananas
½ c unsweetened applesauce (or canned pumpkin)
¼ c nondairy milk
½ tsp vanilla extract
½ tsp bkg soda
1 tsp bkg powder
½ tbsp pumpkin pie spice (or cinnamon)
1 thin slice lemon, with peel (optional)
½ c berries (fresh/frozen) or dried fruit/nuts

Preheat oven to 350°F. Line 8 x 8" pan with parchment paper or use silicon pan. Place oats in bowl. In blender, mix until smooth: bananas, applesauce, milk, vanilla, bkg soda, bkg powder, pumpkin pie spice, and lemon. Fold wet into dry ingredients. Add berries, dried fruit, or nuts. Bake about 23-25 minutes; be careful not to overbake. Cool; cut into bars.

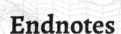

Endnotes

1   Buettner D (2012) *The blue zones: 9 lessons for living longer from the people who've lived the longest.* Washington, DC: National Geographic.

2   Campbell TC, Jacobson H (2013) *Whole: Rethinking the science of nutrition.* Dallas, TX: BenBella Books.

3   *Dietary reference intakes: For energy carbohydrate, fiber, fat, fatty acids, cholesterol, protein, and amino acids.* (2005) Washington, DC: National Academy Press. https://www.nap.edu/read/10490/chapter/1

4   US Department of Agriculture, Agricultural Research Service, Nutrient Data Laboratory. USDA National Nutrient Database for Standard Reference, Release 28. Sept 2015, revised May 2016.

5   Eisman G (2015) *Animal protein and cancer risk.* Lecture presented at North American Vegetarian Society Summerfest, University of Pittsburgh, Johnstown, PA.

6   Physicians Committee for Responsible Medicine (2015) *How can I get enough protein? The protein myth.* Retrieved from http://www.pcrm.org/health/diets/vegdiets/how-can-i-get-enough-protein-the-protein-myth

7   Adventist Health Studies (nd) Retrieved from http://publichealth.llu.edu/adventist-health-studies?rsource=adventisthealthstudy.com

     Greger M (2013) Animal protein and the cancer promoter IGF-1. Retrieved from https://nutritionfacts.org/2013/02/14/animal-protein-and-igf-1

     Ji J, Sundquist J, Sundquist K (2015) Lactose intolerance and risk of lung, breast and ovarian cancers: Aetiological clues from a population-based study in Sweden. *Br J Cancer*, 112(1), 149-52. doi:10.1038/bjc.2014.544

     Tantamango-Bartley Y, Jaceldo-Siegl K, Fan J, Fraser, G (2012) Vegetarian diets and the incidence of cancer in a low-risk population. *Cancer Epidemiology Biomarkers & Prevention, 22(2)*, 286-294. doi:10.1158/1055-9965.epi-12-1060

8   Barnard N (2017) *The cheese trap: How breaking a surprising addiction will help you lose weight, gain energy, and get healthy.* NY, NY: Grand Central Life & Style.

9   Greger M (2014) Do vegetarians get enough protein? Retrieved from https://nutritionfacts.org/video/do-vegetarians-get-enough-protein

10 *AICR eNews* (2015) Retrieved from http://www.aicr.org/enews/2015/06-june

Anand P, Kunnumakkara A, Sundaram C, et al (2008) Cancer is a preventable disease that requires major lifestyle changes. *Pharm Res.* 25(2200). doi:10.1007/s11095-008-9690-4

Anderson M (2009) *Healing cancer from inside out: A practical guide to healing cancer with the rave diet and lifestyle.* RaveDiet.com.

Campbell TC (2017) The past, present, and future of nutrition and cancer: Part 1—was a nutritional association acknowledged a century ago? *Nutrition and Cancer.* doi:10.1080/01635581.2017.1317823

Campbell TC, Jacobson H (2013) *Whole: Rethinking the science of nutrition.* Dallas, TX: BenBella Books.

Greger M (2013) How do plant-based diets fight cancer? Retrieved from https://nutritionfacts.org/2013/02/07/how-do-plant-based-diets-fight-cancer

Irigaray P, Newby JA, Clapp R, et al (2007) Lifestyle-related factors and environmental agents causing cancer: An overview. *Biomed Pharmacother,* 61(10):640-58.

Lodi A, Saha A, Lu X, et al (2017) Combinatorial treatment with natural compounds in prostate cancer inhibits prostate tumor growth and leads to key modulations of cancer cell metabolism. *Precision Oncology.* doi:10.1038/s41698-017-0024-z

11 Greger M (2011) Antioxidant power of plant foods vs. animal foods. Retrieved from https://nutritionfacts.org/video/antioxidant-power-of-plant-foods-versus-animal-foods

12 Greger M (2013) Animal protein and the cancer promoter IGF-1. Retrieved from https://nutritionfacts.org/2013/02/14/animal-protein-and-igf-1

13 Campbell TC, Campbell T (2005) *China study: Startling implications for diet, weight loss and long-term health.* Dallas, TX: BenBella Books. (p.66)

14 McCullough M (2012) The bottom line on soy and breast cancer risk. *American Cancer Society.* Retrieved from http://blogs.cancer.org/expertvoices/2012/08/02/the-bottom-line-on-soy-and-breast-cancer-ris

15 *AICR eNews* (2015) Retrieved from: http://www.aicr.org/enews/2015/06-june/

16 McDougall J (2016) Does sugar feed cancer? *The McDougall Newsletter,* 15(9). Retrieved from https://www.drmcdougall.com/misc/2016nl/sep/sugarcancer.htm

17 Arnold A, Jiang L, Stefanick ML, et al (2016) Duration of adulthood overweight, obesity, and cancer risk in the Women's Health Initiative: A longitudinal study from the United States. *PLoS Med.*

Bazzano LA, Hu T, Reynolds K, et al (2014) Effects of low-carbohydrate and low-fat diets: A randomized trial. *Ann Intern Med.*

Endocrinology S (2017) Breast cancer risk is more affected by total body fat than abdominal fat. *Medical News Today.* Retrieved from http://www.medicalnewstoday.com/releases/317498.php

Kyrgiou M, Kalliala I, Markozanne G, et al (2017) Adiposity and cancer at major anatomical sites: Umbrella review of the literature. *BMJ.*

Sandoiu A (2017) Just one small glass of wine per day increases breast cancer risk. *Medical News Today.* Retrieved from http://www.medicalnewstoday.com/articles/317585.php

18   Greger M (2008) Raw vs. cooked broccoli. Retrieved from http://nutritionfacts.org/video/raw-vs-cooked-broccoli-2

19   Greger M (2010) Best cooking method. Retrieved from http://nutritionfacts.org/video/best-cooking-method

20   *Physicians Committee for Responsible Medicine* (2013) New GEICO study shows how plant-based diets improve nutrition. Retrieved from http://www.pcrm.org/media/online/sep2013/geico-employee-wellness-program-shows-plant-based

21   Campbell TC, Jacobson H (2013) *Whole: Rethinking the science of nutrition.* Dallas, TX: BenBella Books.

22   Greger M (2009) The healthiest sweetener. Retrieved from https://nutritionfacts.org/video/the-healthiest-sweetener

23   Greger M (2012) Erythritol may be a sweet antioxidant. Retrieved from https://nutritionfacts.org/video/erythritol-may-be-a-sweet-antioxidant/

24   Nichols H (2016) Stevia: health benefits, facts, safety. *Medical News Today.* Retrieved from http://www.medicalnewstoday.com/articles/287251.php

25   Greger M (2010) Is stevia good for you? Retrieved from https://nutritionfacts.org/video/is-stevia-good-for-you/

26   Greger M (2009) Forego fat-free dressings? Retrieved from https://nutritionfacts.org/video/forego-fat-free-dressings

27   Servan-Schreiber D (2008) *Anticancer: A new way of life.* NY, NY: Penguin Group. (p 120)

28   Lisle D, Goldhamer A (2006) *The pleasure trap: Mastering the hidden force that undermines health and happiness.* Healthy Living Publications.

29   Barnard N (2007) *Dr. Neal Barnard's program for reversing diabetes: The scientifically proven system for reversing diabetes without drugs.* Emmaus, PA: Rodale Books.

30   Brauser D (2011) Trans-fats linked to increased depression risk. *Medscape.* Retrieved from http://www.medscape.com/viewarticle/736460

Brauser D (2012) Junk food linked to depression. *Medscape*. Retrieved from http://www.medscape.com/viewarticle/762655

Cassels C (2010) Whole diet may ward off depression and anxiety. *Medscape*. Retrieved from http://www.medscape.com/viewarticle/715239

Glynn S (2012) Dieting can lead to food withdrawal and depression. *Medical News Today*. Retrieved from http://www.medicalnewstoday.com/articles/254105.php

Greger M (2015) Plant-based diets for improved mood and productivity. Retrieved from https://nutritionfacts.org/video/plant-based-diets-for-improved-mood-and-productivity

Lucas M, Chocano-Bedoya P, Schulze MB, et al (2014) Inflammatory dietary pattern and risk of depression among women. *Brain Behav Immun*. 36:46-53. doi:10.1016/j.bbi.2013.09.014

McIntosh J (2015) Adhering to a healthy diet could reduce risk of depression. *Medical News Today*. Retrieved from http://www.medicalnewstoday.com/articles/299490.php

University of Warwick (2016) Fruit and veg give you the feel-good factor: New research suggests up to eight-a-day can make you happier. *Medical News Today*. Retrieved from http://www.medicalnewstoday.com/releases/311614.php

Whiteman H (2017) Eating fruits and vegetables may lower women's stress risk. *Medical News Today*. Retrieved from http://www.medicalnewstoday.com/articles/316414.php

31   Karges C (2015) Serotonin, comfort foods and trauma. *Eating Disorder Hope*. Retrieved from https://www.eatingdisorderhope.com/blog/serotonin-comfort-foods-and-trauma

32   Humane Research Council (2014) Study of current and former vegetarians and vegans. Retrieved from spot.humaneresearch.org/2014vegstudy

About the Author

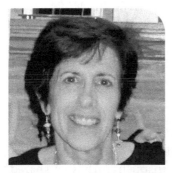

In this book, Sally Lipsky, PhD, combines her expertise in the field of adult learning with her knowledge and passion about plant-based nutrition. During her noteworthy career as a professor of education, Sally authored articles and textbooks on college-level learning and peer-led instruction. A diagnosis of late-stage cancer changed her career path. She began educating herself about the power of food to heal and protect from disease, thereby starting her journey into plant-based eating.

Sally earned a Certificate in Plant-based Nutrition from the T. Colin Campbell Center for Nutrition Studies (delivered by eCornell), completed the Food for Life Program Training (by PCRM), the Farms-to-Forks Weekend Immersion, and the Culinary Rx plant-based wellness course.

Sally currently leads presentations, classes, and workshops on topics related to plant-based nutrition. She's authored articles, a monthly newsletter, and a self-directed curriculum for Physician Assistant students. Sally also is a certified yoga instructor.

Author Contact Information

website: **PlantBasedEatingHub.com**

email: **PlantBasedEatingHub@gmail.com**

Facebook: **PlantBasedEatingHub**

Acknowledgments

My deep appreciation to the people who contributed to the book. To Susan Dawkins, Arden Hamer, Lulu Herold, Kylie Lichtenstein, Lisa Skeers, and Marsha Wong for their valuable feedback. To Marty Howell, Linda Jones, and Roberta Woodfork for sharing their stories and information. And to members of the Pittsburgh East-Suburban Plant-Based Nutrition Support Group who contributed wonderful recipes.

In addition, a heartfelt thank you to Nelson Campbell for his generous and kind foreword.

Finally, my gratitude to the pioneering professionals in the field of whole food, plant-based nutrition. Their integrity and determination, often in the face of deep opposition, are inspiring. They've shared life-changing information so that others, such as myself, can learn and thrive.

Index

CPSIA information can be obtained
at www.ICGtesting.com
Printed in the USA
LVHW02s0045290618
582188LV00012B/1449/P

YOUR FOOD CAN INFLUENCE YOUR CANCER SURVIVAL

A cancer diagnosis is frightening and overwhelming. Standard treatment aside, information on how to fight this disease is confusing and conflicting.

What if you could maximize cancer survival and long-term health just by your diet? In this book, you'll discover:

- What a plant-based diet is and is not
- Why eating plants is crucial to fighting, and preventing, cancer
- Step-by-step guidance for daily plant-centered eating
- How to empower yourself by using food for healing

If you're a cancer survivor, caregiver, or want to prevent cancer, this book gives you practical steps to eat for long-term health, including:

- Resources for eating nutritionally and conveniently
- Tips for creating healthy eating habits
- Practical advice for restaurants, travel, and social events
- Tasty, yet simple recipes

Sally Lipsky, a late-stage cancer survivor, has a Ph.D. in education and decades of teaching experience. She spent years researching how to survive and thrive with cancer and is living proof that it's possible.

This book guides you step-by-step as you begin your plant-based journey to healing and peace of mind.

Success stories from cancer survivors:

Plant-based eating has become a delicious and nutritious venture for me. My doctors are amazed that I'm in such great shape.
— Roberta, breast cancer survivor

When I learned about plant-based eating, I was surprised how delicious the food was. By 2013, I'd lost much weight, gotten off blood pressure medication, and completed a sprint triathlon! I never felt better.
— Marty, late-stage colon cancer survivor

HEALTH
CANCER

ISBN 9781988645056

90000 >

9 781988 645056

HOW TO BECOME YOUR OWN ODYSSEY,
OR | THE LAND OF INDIGESTION

Edmund Wong woke early on Saturday to gray skies, the San Francisco weather that made his bedroom door stick and the window fog up. He felt anxious for the warmth that surrounded his mother after she woke up the kitchen: coffee boiling on the stove, just-washed dishes steaming on the rack beside the sink, the glowing half-light of morning.

He bounded down the stairs in his flannel pajamas and nearly tripped over his father sleeping on the kitchen floor—one arm curled under his head and the other soaking in a puddle of sesame oil. Mrs. Wong stood over her husband, hand cradling her pregnant belly. She turned to her son. "Edmund, I don't know where your dad is trying to go," she said in Cantonese.

Edmund didn't look away from his snoring father, whose eyes were wide open. He knew that his mother, in her turquoise terry-cloth robe, sash tied crookedly over her bulging middle, had followed his father around their darkened house late last night; that she'd waddled ahead to move chairs and push sharp table corners out of her husband's path. And in the early morning light, unable to ever leave a mess when she found one, she had wiped big greasy handprints off the kitchen walls and counters.

Edmund's mother poked his father's arm with her toe. "When your dad sleepwalks, he gets sleep-hungry. Ai-ya! His appetite. Everything into his mouth—whole tofu blocks, raw cabbage, even radishes. And your dad *hates* radishes." She absentmindedly rubbed her protruding stomach.

"Why'd you leave him here?" Edmund crouched next to his father, who had stopped snoring, and put a finger to his nose to make sure that he was still breathing. "What if something happens to him?"

"You're only nine. Why do you worry like an old man?"

Edmund could not read his mother's expression. Her tone was not of concern; rather, it held the same resolve as when Edmund's father lost his job as the manager of a small antiques shop, and Mrs. Wong had to struggle to keep a roof over their heads. Edmund had been just six at the time and did not understand what the word *embezzlement* meant, or what it had to do with losing their home and moving into the damp cottage behind old Mr. Moon's house. But even at six, he understood why the antiques dealer, a seventy-year-old woman named Mrs. Bahn, did not turn his father in to the police. Edmund still dreamed of the picnics Mrs. Bahn had packed for antiques hunting trips with the Wongs: baskets filled with fragrant pickled cabbage, plump red grapes, and icy bottles of saké that made the adults laugh and talk for hours while Edmund dozed in the shade of a tree or dug holes in the grass in search of worms.

Edmund believed that Mrs. Bahn thought of Mrs. Wong as her adopted daughter; Edmund's mother had that effect on the seniors she spent her time with—like Mrs. Bahn and Mr. Moon—endearing herself to them with her large wide-set eyes that crinkled in the corners when she smiled, her no-nonsense attitude, her sharp mind, her persistent optimism through hardships.

Edmund yearned for those days before his mother found a full-time position as a music teacher at the community college, when money was still very tight because of Mr. Wong's unemployment, a time when Mrs. Wong had to trade piano lessons for rent. Their sympathetic landlord visited the Wongs' cottage and played the same simplistic song over and over, every Tuesday, for months. Edmund knew the landlord never practiced, that the uncoordinated plunking sounds filling their diminutive living room were that of a lonely widower desperate to spend time within the rich folds of Edmund's family.

"Dad's sleepwalking will stop, right? After—" Edmund pointed to his mother's stomach.

"Each time, I hope that he'll wake up and see how stupid he looks, walking around like a zombie." She suddenly squeezed her eyes shut.

"What's wrong?"

"A little kicking." She rubbed her belly again. "Yes, I think your dad will stop when *she's* here. He did when *you* were born." Mom patted where Edmund imagined his sister's head was. "She's telling me the time is near."

Mr. Wong woke, groggy and stiff, just as Edmund finished heating soy milk on the stove. The son peppered his father with questions as he poured the steaming liquid into mugs for himself and his parents. "Well? Well? What did you see? What did you do? Where did you go this time?"

"What can I tell you?" Mr. Wong responded in a husky voice as he sat up and rubbed the sleep out of his eyes. Edmund tossed a gray dish towel to his father, who dabbed at the bright orange sesame oil staining his pajama sleeve. Edmund tried to catch his mother's eye, but she was busy searching through the fridge for the leftover rice porridge. He listened to her mutter as she straddled the pile of shredded uncooked wonton skins and chicken bone splinters and the half-chewed pork dumplings that his father had strewn all over the floor at the base of the fridge.

"Helen," Mr. Wong said to his wife, who was now kneeling, digging through the lowest shelf in search of her breakfast. "Helen," he said a little louder when Mrs. Wong did not respond. "Let Edmund find it for you."

Nudged by his father, Edmund got up and crossed the kitchen, helped his mother stand, put his hands on her shoulders and guided her to a chair. While Edmund stirred the rice porridge on the stove, his mother stretched out her legs, resting her feet on the seat of Edmund's empty chair, her mug of soy milk balanced on top of her stomach. Edmund let the porridge simmer, turned to his father. "Tell me what you saw."

Mr. Wong studied the spot on the floor where the tiles were black and white and glittering, the grout stained orange from the sesame-oil spill. "At night outside it is dark for you," he began, "but when I sleepwalk, there is no difference between night and day."

"I love it! That's awesome!"

"Yeah, yeah, yeah. No difference," Mr. Wong responded, matter-of-factly. "But I don't say that it's awesome or that it's good. Nothing like that."

"Oh?"

Mr. Wong gave his son a placating smile. "I've told you many times, Edmund. The stars and moon shine all the time, not just at night."

"How?" Edmund asked.

"*Plasma*. It's glowing plasma we're seeing."

"*Plas-ma*," Edmund repeated slowly.

His father sighed, then examined the orange towel. "*Most* people see only half the light. Just the sun. It's no wonder they sleep in the dark, sleep without seeing, sleep without going anywhere." He reclined in his chair, closed his eyes, a vague smile on his face. "The moon shines for me, lights my dreams, lights my day and night. I can taste and feel, walk and see in my dreams. I see rivers. I catch fish and ducks with my bare hands. I eat everything."

Edmund nodded vigorously, even though his father couldn't see him. Mr. Wong played with his oily sleeve, then lifted his fingers to his nose. Did they smell like toasted sesames? Or did they smell earthy, salty, like river and algae and fish?

"I don't go to sleep to find the river. The river finds me. I find the answers, always, see everything right in front of me as clearly as the sun." Mr. Wong's voice was suddenly thick and full of phlegm. He curled his greasy fingers into a fist, as if trying to conceal something in his palm. He yawned, then stood, pushing his chair back with a loud scrape, and touched his wife's shoulder. He crossed the kitchen, then knelt stiffly before the fridge. As he began to pick up apple cores and watermelon rinds and shrimp tails, his son stared out through the kitchen window.

Edmund—who spied a seagull flying way up high, a slender black shadow sliding across the flat white sky—wondered: Could birds sleep and fly at the same time, too?

Edmund figured that the easiest way to find answers was to follow his father while he sleepwalked. At dinner, he announced, "Tonight, I will find out where Dad goes."

Mrs. Wong studied her son over her plate of gingery fish and scallops, pickled duck web and salted squid, and bowl of steaming rice. "Edmund," she said, "you sleep like you are dead. Your dad sleeps like he is awake. Do you really think you can follow him?"

"I am one hundred percent positive. I have a plan."

Mrs. Wong shook her head. "Look, last night I followed your dad because he's making a mess in my kitchen. I tell him, 'Wake up! Go back to sleep!' but he just sleepwalks away." She looked up at the ceiling, exhaled loudly and shrugged her shoulders with a sort of amused resignation. Mrs. Wong had fallen in love with her husband because of his desire to make everything he did or said into an Event or a Story. A shoelace breaking became a Story. Boiling the perfect egg became an Event. Every day he brought a sense of drama and excitement to her life. She'd found over the years, however, that this could be exhausting. She often thought about the year before she met her husband; she'd been twenty-two, her first year out of music college, her first year living on her own.

She rented a room from a retired firewoman, Mrs. Garcia. There was nothing in her room except a desk, a chair, a twin bed, and a bookshelf. It was perfect. She'd brought with her a single suitcase that contained all her clothes, one extra pair of shoes, two books, and a thick binder filled with sheets of music scribbled with her notes. Later, she would go to the bookstore and buy a few more books to fill out at least one shelf; she would go to the department store and buy a new dress to wear for auditions. But on that first day, she had almost nothing. She remembered looking out her rented window, seeing the bright blue sky and the top of an oak tree, and down below, the spot on the sidewalk where she'd once stood in front of old Mrs. Garcia's house, wondering which window would be hers. Mrs. Wong had not yet had to compete with Mr. Wong's glamorous sleepwalking stories, his persistent need for an audience, his desire to prove how special his own body was in comparison with his pregnant wife's. She had still been living her own life inside her own orderly little room, when the only audience she wanted was her bold reflection in the bright window.

Mr. Wong twirled a wooden chopstick between his fingers like a baton. "Like I told your mom, you can try to follow me, but these are *my* dreams. I can't just write you instructions, draw you a map, make you a key." He pointed at his temple with his chopstick, then twisted it as if he were using a skeleton key to unlock his mind. "When I sleepwalk, I see things and go where no one else can. Do you understand, Edmund?"

Edmund frowned and watched his mother hungrily scoop out a fish cheek with her spoon. The purple bags under her eyes were more pronounced than they had been in the morning. Her long hair was tangled, her shirt sleeve stained. Questions and concerns that had simmered in the back of Edmund's mind began to boil over: Why wasn't his father afraid of his wife accidentally hurting the baby while she moved furniture out of his way in the darkness? Did his father mean it when he referred to the baby as *an accident* after finishing an entire box of wine the night his mother shared the news? Was he, Edmund, an accident, too?

Later, in bed, Edmund stayed awake for as long as he could, imagining all the things his father had seen the night before: ducks, fish, river water—all bathed in light. He imagined finding his father in the dark living room, watching as he opened a heavy oak door, a golden glow spilling in. He imagined the sounds of water lapping against a worn wooden dock, birds' friendly quacking. And he imagined his father holding the door open for him and his mother, waving them into his dream world, safe from the dangers of birth, from purple eye-bags, from stained sleeves and pinched brows. A world where drunk fathers did not jokingly refer to a child as The Accident: 意外 Edmund pulled the covers up over his chin, rubbed his feet together to get them warm, and slept the sleep of the dead.

Sunday morning Edmund found his mother standing in their driveway, shoulders slumped, hand slowly circling her belly. Mr. Wong was asleep on top of the family's old Chrysler station wagon; his salt-and-pepper hair needed a good combing, and his orange pajama sleeve, which was snagged at the base of the car's antenna, had lost its oily sheen.

Mrs. Wong told her son that the sheets of bubble wrap he'd placed on the floor beside their bed last night *had* popped when Mr. Wong got up. "They sounded just like firecrackers, rat-tat-tat!" she said with full-moon eyes. "But you and your dad still didn't wake up. Only me."

"And the cup of water?" Edmund asked.

"When he pushed open our door, it tipped and splashed *all* over him, just like you planned. He didn't even blink, just smiled. Your dad must have dreamed he was the dragonhead in the Chinese New Year parade. You know how it rains every year." Mrs. Wong mimicked a slithering dragon with her arms. Edmund wondered what the neighbors would think if they saw her, both arms undulating overhead, her robe straining to stay closed over her bulging stomach.

Edmund jabbed a small dirt mound beside the driveway with his slippered toe, then rested it there until ants began to crawl up his leg. He brushed them off and thought about the time he'd left a dead mouse on the ant hill, how he returned each day to see what the ants would do. In just one week, the insects had devoured and carried away the mouse's meat, tendons, cartilage, callused paw pads, fur, even its long gray whiskers. All that remained was the animal's tiny skeleton.

Later that morning, Mr. Wong poured himself a cup of coffee and sat with his son at the table. Edmund pushed aside his unfinished bowl of corn flakes to ask his father about his dreams.

"Tell me! What was it like?"

"They just took me, lifted me with their tremendous wings," said Mr. Wong, who went on to describe the grand forest he'd visited, the spires of trees, the golden-winged creatures that resembled enormous seahorses soaring through the air. "And we went in search of grasslands to stomp on with our hooves. And the feasts we had! Oh, the green garbanzos that glittered like emeralds. Slices of cake the size of . . . of . . . your bed. I just buried my face in frosty clouds of sugar icing. There were prisons, churches, schools . . . built out of bright vermilion pomegranate skins. The red, it was so red. Like a beating heart—."

"Take me with you. Why can't I go?"

"—And then I wake up with dirty feet," continued Mr. Wong, ignoring his son's question. "And my bones creak like a broken wagon wheel, my mouth burns, and my stomach is full, and I know . . . I know that I've been *somewhere*."

"Do you want to listen to my dream?" Edmund asked excitedly. He couldn't actually remember his own dream, so he made up one about a boy swinging on a swing so high that his toes sizzled in the sun. His father's eyes seemed to glaze as he fidgeted with the hem of his shirt. Edmund felt hurt by this; he loved how his mother, unlike Mr. Wong, listened so intently—head tilted in concentration, eyes wide as the boy described the heat of the flame, the meaty crackle of his toenails, the melted rubber of his slippers.

"You can teach me to sleepwalk," said Edmund to his father.

"This is not something you teach." Mr. Wong sighed.

"Why? I don't get it! Why?" asked Edmund. What he really wanted to ask was whether his father preferred his sun-drenched dreaming life to his awake life with a son and wife. Did his father feel caged in? When he slumbered his way to their station wagon, was he trying to leave his family? When he chewed cantaloupe rinds, raw shrimp, whole sticks of butter, was he trying to fill his insides with his dream life?

Weighed down by his need to understand, Edmund felt his questions turn to rocks in his own stomach. "Why don't you believe in me?"

Mr. Wong closed his eyes. For a long time, he just sat there, slowly breathing in and out, oblivious. Edmund could not tell if his father was awake or asleep.

That night, as soon as Edmund's parents went to bed, he snuck down to the kitchen. Unlike in the morning, when the room glowed with his mother's light, the space was inky black. Edmund's footsteps were muffled by his thick socks and the hum of the refrigerator; the floor felt sticky. Edmund approached the pantry, pulled out boxes of waffle mix, week-old brownies, a bag of sesame seeds, molasses, a jar of canola oil, a can of garbanzo beans, a bag of flour. He hunted through the fridge and grabbed celery, spinach dip, an enormous bunch of bok choy, milk. In his hushed hunger, he crunched into the celery and bok choy with his fangs. He inhaled handfuls of seeds, which he washed down with milk and garbanzo juice. He peeled the plastic lid off the tub of dip, spread the creamy paste on slices of bread, sprinkled beans on top, then stuffed it all into his mouth. He waded into the bag of flour like a dusty moth, grabbed fistfuls to mix with canola oil and dark brown molasses. He shoveled the mud down his throat.

After what felt like hours, Edmund stood back to view his progress. The muck on his hands had hardened into a thick glove; when he wiggled his fingers, the crust crumbled. The air swirled with flour. Bags and boxes and empty cans were strewn around the kitchen. Edmund had barely made a dent in the food, yet his stomach churned and bellowed. He marveled at how his mother could carry all this weight, this rich, roiling life inside of her, for nine whole months. His stomach pinched again, and he wished right then that he could die, that his parents would find him, carry his body down to the ant hill. He wished for the small mound to turn into a great peak, for ants the size of salamanders to peel his body apart and march away with his meat, his arms and hips and thighs, devour him all the way down, clear to the bone.

Edmund left his mess, crept back to his bed without washing up. He rubbed his stomach and, as he fell asleep, thought about how he was no longer just his father's fragile shadow, just residue biology. Edmund wanted to tell his father to not be scared of the new baby, to look at how he (Edmund) had become his own odyssey, journeyed to the land of indigestion without maps or charts, and the ground was vibrating just for him.

Sometime after midnight, a jolt sent Edmund tumbling out of bed, his sheets wrapped around him like he was a pork dumpling. With his cheek smashed against the floor, he listened to the earthquake; it cracked and rumbled and let out a deep boom like thunder. The oak floorboards rolled, and water sloshed out of Ed Junior Junior's fish tank.

"This is the big one!" the boy yelled.

Strong arms slid around him. His mother. She grabbed him, sheets and all, and bolted out to the backyard. By the time they reached the bench in the center of the garden, the shaking had stopped and Edmund was wide awake.

He was shocked to find his father already seated on the bench in his white pajamas, head cranked back, chin and slow-blinking brown eyes aimed at the night sky. Had his father sleepwalked himself to safety just before the earthquake hit, leaving behind his family? Edmund wrapped the sheets tighter around himself and pressed in close. He wanted his father to pat his head or squeeze his shoulder, but Mr. Wong just continued to breathe, evenly and heavily, out of his gaping mouth.

A baby cried somewhere nearby, and shouts echoed up and down their street, dark from the power outage. While Mrs. Wong dug around in their small, messy toolshed in search of a flashlight, Edmund followed his father's gaze. It was a clear night; the earthquake must have shaken all the fog away. The moon, white and shaped like a watermelon slice, peeked out from just over the neighbor's house. Was the moon scared, too?

The whole sky seemed to grow smaller as it moved up and away, to make room for the stars burning in the blue-black horizon. Unlike the moon, the stars were not hiding. There were thousands of shimmering clusters, and behind those were millions more. The longer Edmund stared, the more stars appeared. He was afraid that the darkness could not hold so much light, and the stars would fall like fiery apples from a tree, right onto their heads.

Mrs. Wong returned with an enormous flashlight, which she carried snug against her side like a loaf of bread. "No batteries. Ai-ya! What does your dad do when he's not sleeping?" She squeezed her husband's shoulder, gave him a little shake. When he did not stir, Mrs. Wong exhaled loudly. Edmund wondered if the next night, his mother might leave the station wagon door unlocked, keep the key in the ignition for his father.

Mrs. Wong looked up at the slowly rising moon and breathed in deeply the cold night air. "Remember this sky, Edmund," she said in the tone of someone who had unlocked all the world's secrets, of someone whose feet were always planted heavily, firmly, on the juddering ground. "You might never see it like this again."

When Edmund offered to return to the house to find a working flashlight, his mother responded, "I'll get it. Stay with him." Mrs. Wong pointed to her husband. "He needs you."

Edmund stayed put, though he did not know what his father could possibly need from him. Mrs. Wong started to stand, but the baby kicked her painfully in the ribs. She winced, sat back down, and rubbed her stomach.

"Edmund, you will have to go get the batteries," said Mrs. Wong. She tilted her head as she listened for the creaking of the house's brittle walls, or for any signs that the structure might be too dangerous to return to. She handed her son the useless flashlight.

Edmund pulled off the bedsheet, then draped the fuzzy orange flannel around his mother's shoulders.

Mr. Wong sighed loudly and smacked his lips like he was hungry, and Edmund suddenly understood what his mother meant about his father needing him. He cringed when he thought about his mother tripping over the mess he'd left in the kitchen earlier, and vowed never to stuff himself that way again. He thought of his father's grand, dreamed-up stories, the way that he sprawled on the hood of the car and on the kitchen floor for everyone to find him in the morning. He thought about the way his mother, though deep into her pregnancy, felt compelled to clean up Mr. Wong's deranged banquets. Recalling how he'd begged his father to take him on his sleepwalking journeys, Edmund shook his head; how could someone take so much, yet give so little? He wanted to pluck a star from the sky and put it in his father's mouth so that he lit up from the inside out. Then light would shine from his father's eyeballs, and mouth, and even his ears, so he could guide his family always to safety.

Mrs. Wong smiled as Edmund trotted toward the house, the flashlight clutched in hand, periodically stopping to look up at the sky and exclaim softly, breathlessly, "Wow." She felt a mixed sense of pride and trepidation as she witnessed her son brave the dark, do what her husband could not do, and venture where he could not see.

LITTLE HARLOT

Clatter of chopsticks, rice bowls on wobbly folding tables we'd draped in our best linens, smacking lips of aunties and uncles greedily eating our best food: roasted pig pieces, oily duck chunks, creamy yellow macaroni-and-cheese casserole, platters of chicken-shawarma-stuffed pita, and paper-thin chocolatey slivers of Grandma's favorite Mars bars for dessert.

The baby, hidden under a heart-print blanket Lin had strung around her chest with a shoelace, makes kissing sounds like the couples do in the movies I'd recently started to watch. My eighteen-year-old cousin was Mama's cautionary tale: "That harlot. Sex in a station wagon. All those stains."

The first time I'd heard this story, I was seven. I didn't know what the word *harlot* meant and believed that Mama was upset with Lin for leaving stains in the car (like the time I'd spilt a liter of grape soda on the sofa). I loved the way *harlot* sounded, the breathiness of the hard *h*, the brittle *t*, and the snap of the tongue against the roof of my mouth as I finished saying the mighty word. I had walked around for days after hearing Lin's story, calling everyone I admired, everyone I believed to be brave (like the kid at school who cussed out a mean teacher), a *harlot*.

A loud crash in the kitchen.

"Grandma, we're glad you're visiting us. But don't let us see you!" shouts B-actress auntie, rubber-gasket heiress, mouth full, oily smears on her lips.

Lin rolls her eyes. I ask Lin who the daddy is.

"No one." Lin hands me the baby and joins in at the tables. I lay the baby across my legs, gently squeeze and rub together the folds of fat on her stomach until they turn pink, as if they are two halves of a squishy steamed bun. The baby doesn't even flinch. I am enthralled with the tough little harlot. I lift her, blow on the strawberry pinch. The vibrations tickle my nose. I bury my face in the baby's tuft of head hair, inhale deeply the scent of her scalp, place my hand on her round belly, feel quick bird breaths, warmth, under soiled yellow terry cloth.

I think of when Grandma died: early morning darkness, Mama seated at the edge of my bed, whispering to me, voice gravelly with grief. She tells of finding Grandma in her favorite chair, kitten tightly curled on her lap. Grandma did not have a cat, but I didn't correct Mama when she described the animal's rough tongue licking furiously, as though rasping life from Grandma's translucent skin.

I imagine the story kitten, small as a fist, brown as a paper bag, with x's for eyes, tongue dangling. I imagine it circling three times, tiny claws piercing Grandma's thin skin through cotton pajamas, a furry ball in the dent between Grandma's bony legs. Did Grandma's last breaths sound like a ragged purr?

Lin returns. I watch her struggle with the baby sling. I remain silent, small as the D&D orc miniature I'd stored in my pocket, intending to trade with another cousin. The baby observes the ceiling, as if searching for answers to a difficult question.

We weave between aunties and uncles wavering on their feet, drunk on funeral wine. We push between cousins, inhaling their pungent scent of deodorant and onion. I step on the toe of an uncle who is busy collecting used cups and plates in a square plastic tub that Dad uses to soak his feet. From across the room, my parents wave tiredly at me, captains on Grandma's drunken boat funeral tour. I do not wave back.

Upstairs, sweat beads my upper lip. I wipe it away like a cowboy. Lin strolls into a room, picks a glittering brooch out of a relative's suitcase, holds it to the light. Rolls a gold pen between fingers, touches it with the tip of her tongue. Finds an unopened bag of sour-apple rings, rips it wide, stuffs two of the candies in her mouth before offering me some. Then flips open an uncle's diary, made of sturdy cowhide, with sketches of copper mountains, golden clouds, words of sadness. Lin inhales deeply, the leather, ink, and gilded grief.

The baby faces outward from the sling on Lin's chest; she reaches for red wool socks, silky panties, opal-faced lighters with mesmerizing blue flames. My cousin and I sniff, probe, lick our way through our relatives' belongings. Before Lin opens each door, she turns, puts a finger to her lips. "Shhhhh."

We make our way to my parents' bedroom. In Mama's jewelry box, a heavy jade ring, pearl earrings, a diamond cat pin. I observe the pile of black polyester dresses Mama tried on before dinner. I know my parents would use their favorite American phrase if they caught us snooping through our family's luggage: *Didn't anyone tell you that curiosity killed the cat?*

Lin angrily rummages. "Why does she need all of this?"

I don't know how to respond, so I busy myself with folding Mama's dresses and pretend that I didn't hear.

"Why do people keep so much crap they don't even like, when they know other people could use it?" she asks.

I've eavesdropped on enough of Mama's phone conversations to know that Lin had been a freshman in college, and seven months pregnant, when she gave up her full scholarship and dropped out of a prestigious biology program. She'd moved back into her parents' small cottage located on a fallow orchard—a three-hour train ride from the university—to have her baby. Mama and I once visited Lin and her family. I still think of the depressing grassy expanse surrounding their home. I think of the quail, small brown birds who'd eaten the fermented fruit rotting on the ground below desiccated peach trees, how the birds tottered drunkenly around the orchard, slamming into one another as they ran away from me.

I watch Lin try to jam her feet into Mama's taupe suede pumps, which are clearly two sizes too small for my cousin. She removes them, studies the unworn leather soles, frowns. Lin's family had struggled during the time surrounding her pregnancy; after paying back the scholarship to the university, they'd had to sell their meager belongings to make ends meet. And when they had nothing left to sell, they asked for loans from relatives. My parents had tried to gift them money, but Lin's father stubbornly refused to accept any charity. Mama had remarked that Lin never forgave her parents for selling her biology textbooks.

The baby sucks a frayed bra strap. I finger one of Mama's delicate gold-plated chains, lick—taste of a paperclip—then put it back.

"Take something," says Lin, who's stopped digging through Mama's drawer of synthetic silk stockings. "Really. I want to give you something." She slips on Mama's jade ring, a coveted heirloom inherited from Grandma. Something stirs in me as I watch Lin buff the enormous jade cabochon using the fabric of the baby's sling. Maybe it's watching her clean something that's not hers, but I have the urge to give Mama's precious ring to Lin. I want my cousin to wear its luxe weight on her finger. I want the brilliant green to contrast with Lin's intense brown eyes. I want Lin to have Mama's and Grandma's years of good luck. But how do you take something that isn't yours? And even more perplexing: How do you *give* something that isn't yours?

I look to the baby, who is kicking the air in her dreams. Thick drool glimmers around her mouth. I wonder at my cousin's bravery for carrying this ferocious, punting human inside of her. Lin uses a silk scarf and wipes the wetness from the baby's chin.

"Why'd you do it?" I point to the baby.

"I've captured glowing bugs before," Lin responds, seemingly ignoring my question. "Well, not really bugs. They're called dino-flagellates . . . plankton. It's bioluminescence. Do you know what that is? Did you know we have those?"

I shake my head.

"For a school project, I went and caught these things, like teensy, almost microscopic, animals."

"How teensy?"

"So small. They float around in the bay. Imagine thousands of them coming together, these incredible blue-green clouds that glow in the water at night. And when fish chase after them, the clouds swirl and glow even brighter. And then herons come—these grand black birds—to chase after the fish. It becomes like this whole universe of stars underwater, shimmering shimmering shimmering. It's quite spectacular." Lin walks across the room, drops the ring into an empty vase with a loud clang. My eyes dart to the doorway. I listen for footsteps.

"Anyway, I kept some in water in an old applesauce jar. These beautiful shimmering things."

"Do you still have them?"

Lin shrugs, drops Mama's earrings into the same vase. Curiously, I feel relieved knowing that the ring will not be alone, that like the glowing bugs, the earrings and ring will rattle around the bottom of the vase together.

I wonder if Lin kept the jar in her stained station wagon. I imagine the daytime heat inside her car, the dirty jar water. I wonder what she fed them. I picture glowing bugs floating to the surface on sour-apple-ring life preservers, trying to suck air through tiny punctures in the lid.

"I know people see me as some harlot. I'm not deaf. I hear them on the phone—like your *mom*—talking to my parents, calling me this word." Lin's brows are knitted, her brown eyes fixed on me when she asks, "What do you think? Do you think I'm a harlot?"

My cheeks flush. My throat closes, and I cannot speak.

Lin continues, "When I finally told my boyfriend about the baby, he wanted me to quit school, said, 'Babies. What more do you need to know about biology?' He said that I didn't need to learn anything else, that nothing outside of our family should matter. My parents said the same thing. Everyone said the same thing. That I should quit school. But why should I quit this world? They all said their love was enough for me, for us." She kisses the top of the baby's head. "But what'd they do for me that I wasn't already doing for myself?" Lin takes a deep breath, strokes the downy hairs atop the baby's head. "I think . . . I wish I'd found another way. I wish that I'd defied them all, showed them, and stayed in school."

I am silent, terrified of saying the wrong thing. I look into her eyes, then over at the baby, who is sleeping with her tiny fist shoved into her mouth. And I realize that the ring would never have been enough for Lin. I don't know what would have been, what answer might help Lin to hear the word *harlot* in the way that I first did, as a term of strength, defiance, independence. I want to ask her what she is looking for when she snoops through Mama's belongings, when she eats just a few pieces of someone else's candy and then leaves the torn bag, when she moves jewelry around someone's room without pocketing anything, or reads someone else's diary without revealing its secrets—what is she looking for, and why does she not take what she needs?

The sleeping baby punches the air in her dreams; I wonder about her first words, what she'll have to say. Will she stand up for Lin, tight little fists swinging at anyone calling her mother a harlot? Will she align with my miniature orc—tough, loud-mouthed, a survivor even if some call it evil?

I feel something like pride, as Lin's cousin, when I picture Lin proving everyone wrong: attending biology classes, peering into a microscope while teaching her lab partner about dinoflagellates and all their shimmer, Lin's baby in a sling on her back, chugging milk out of an Erlenmeyer flask.

Lin uses one of Mama's dresses to wipe her nose. "Life is not just living for another person." She takes a shuddering breath, stands.

I am reminded of what Mama had said when I asked how she could go out to dinner with Baba just days after Grandma's passing: "Ellie, it is survival. You can't go around feeling shame for living. You can't stop your own journey simply because someone else's deviates or has come to an end. Accepting what I cannot change, that my life matters and is my own, *that* is how I can honor your grandma."

As I watch Lin struggle to pull one of Mama's rings off her fat thumb, I begin to wonder why Mama and the other adults couldn't honor Lin this way, allowing my cousin to live her life in her own way, to take her own path. I try to imagine being Lin—ridiculed by aunties and pushed by my parents into believing that a child should replace my other dreams, when being a mother was both too much and not enough. A life being called a name I hated, whispers following me everywhere like an angry shadow.

Lin pulls from her pocket a pair of white silk panties harvested from one of the aunties' suitcases. "Look what I found." She does a squirming dance as she pulls them on under her skirt. The baby, jostled awake, cries loudly. "Isn't this a thrill?" exclaims Lin over the racket. "I'm going to wear them. I'm gonna stain the hell out of 'em. Our secret. Will you tell?"

THE RICHMOND

I hated where we lived in San Francisco's Richmond District, three blocks from the Pacific Ocean, two blocks from the community center with its low ceilings and dreary salt-scrubbed façade. I hated the Richmond's brackish air, its June fog when everywhere else felt like real summer. I hated my middle school, which boasted of its only claim to fame—a contest to see who could wear shorts all summer long—in its annual newsletter.

"Mama, why can't we just move to a better district?" I asked on the last day of sixth grade. I was eleven, my hands stuffed into my pockets. We were waiting for our bus to take us home, watching the rich kids get into their parents' cars.

Mama ignored my question. Instead, she waved at a mom she recognized, who was driving in a car headed for the special math-and-science summer camp that offered its pupils brand-name sodas and brand-name futures. The mom had shiny black curls that reminded me of Mrs. Wan, one of my parents' oldest friends, who curled her hair to abandon. I pictured both Mrs. Wan and the woman from the car sleeping in hard plastic curlers, waking with tender scalps each morning.

The woman's daughter, the sixth-grade class president, stuck her tongue out at me through the open car window as they drove past. I stared at my shoes, wishing to disappear. Mama turned to study my face, her eyes brown and puzzled. She didn't look toward the street when a driver in another car honked at someone. She didn't point out the stain on my shirt from my cranberry juice box. When she spoke, she did so quietly and firmly. "What do people know?" she said. "Having more money doesn't mean anything if you don't know how to keep your tongue from falling out of your head."

I pushed Mama's kindness away with a violent shake of my head. I didn't know how to tell her that it wasn't the tongue wagging in the wind I was upset about. It was Mrs. Waterson, a substitute food-slinger, a white woman with silvering hair and shriveled arms who'd filled in for our beloved cafeteria manager, Mr. Gonzalez.

"Do. You. Want. A. Scoop. Of. This?" Mrs. Waterson had asked the student before me in line, a shy eighth-grade Chinese girl with a purple birthmark the size of a hand on her right cheek. "Do. You. Want. Po-ta-toes?" she enunciated, her volume turned up just slightly.

When the eighth grader declined, Mrs. Waterson turned her syrupy smile to me, the same scoop of dreary, off-white mashed potatoes stretched out in front of her. "How. About. You? Do. You. Want. Potatoes?"

My cheeks flushed, my hands clenched the plastic tray, and I could feel my heart pounding in my ears. I didn't know what was happening to me. All I knew was that Mrs. Waterson had not spoken like this to the two white kids who'd gone ahead of us in line, and the change in the old woman's voice cut through me.

In my dreams now, I often return to that moment. It is once again 1970. I am eleven years old. But in the dreams I understand what ignorance looks and sounds like. I have the language to describe that feeling of being singled out, of needing to constantly prove my worth, my humanity. I am eleven and I understand that the poison that comes out of our mouths can hurt us more than the dreary potatoes we put in. That these tiny humiliations can fissure rooms, separate the spaces: one for Belonging, one for Not Belonging. It can stamp invisible passports that give only certain people the freedom to inhabit the world without question, allow these same people to be the default everyone else is compared to. They call out your name, slowly, deliberately, with a smile that cleaves you in two.

"Why do we live *here*?" I asked Mama again. I gestured around at the gray sidewalk, the seagull droppings that stained the concrete. What I really wanted to know was whether I'd ever make it to the sheltered heart of our city—a place I imagined like the lost city of Atlantis, a place I wasn't sure even existed, so circumscribed were our lives. I imagined a golden school with grand basketball courts and libraries, with no math tests, with teachers and kids who looked and sounded like me. And where it was never foggy. There were crisp blue skies, wide and open and full of possibilities.

Mama looked hard at me for a moment, then up into the tangled black web of trolley cables that choked the sky overhead. "What do you mean *here*, Mei?" she asked, brushing a strand of hair out of my face.

I winced, imagining how Mrs. Waterson would have spoken to Mama if she'd heard her accent.

"Why do you always have to take everything so personally?" Mama continued. "You're not going to survive if you don't know how to just . . . shake it off when someone sticks their tongue out at you. She'll grow up."

"Is this all you want for me? This school, the stupid rich kids who get everything?" I said. "Mrs. Waterson?"

"Who is this Mrs. Waterson?"

I frowned, crossed my arms over my chest. The bus arrived, and we sat in silence until we reached the stop in front of our apartment.

"Mei?" asked Mama as she opened the front door with her jangle of keys. I didn't know what to say. But when she placed a plate of my favorite after-school snack—smudges of blended chicken liver smeared onto large square whole-grain crackers—my resolve finally snapped, and the story about Mrs. Waterson spilled out. Mama listened as she finished the dishes, her fingers pruned. She wiped her hands on her apron and sat down beside me.

"I'm so proud of you for sharing this with me," she began. "These things . . . I cannot tell you that these things will not happen to you again."

"Why can't we go somewhere we don't have to deal with people like her?"

"You think that it's *better* outside of the Richmond?" Mama's voice was slightly raised, her cheeks pink. "You leave here, then where would you go?"

Since I didn't know how to describe my Atlantis, I said the only other place that came to mind, "Chinatown," though I only visited there once each year, and just briefly to stop at the only bakery in the city that made their lotus seed cake without the inferior white kidney bean paste.

"Chinatown? It's not so easy. We move to Chinatown, and you think they won't tease you for speaking Chinese with an American accent? For being born here? For being *too* American? Or that they won't look down on me for raising you in all this?" She gestured around at our tiny kitchen. Following the path of her arm, my gaze stuck on the pair of shears with razor-sharp teeth that she used to cut whole chicken carcasses in half.

I'd always known that Mama and Baba refused to leave our foggy little Chinese hamlet. Though my parents had traveled here from across the world—me smaller than a twig inside Mama's uterus when they first arrived in the States—now they would no longer go east of Arguello Boulevard unless it was for special desserts. I'd thought this was because our area was filled with all the top-notch vegetable markets, gossipy fishmongers, and bustling

Chinese restaurants serving cow's throat tendon, pork dumplings, cloud-ear fungus, hotpots overflowing with steamy, bubbling chicken broth. Where each Sunday morning, Mama and Baba proudly stalked the streets, hunting for bargains among other Chinese couples—packs of silver- and black-haired people wearing the same sensible flat sneakers, the same unfussy jackets and lumpy hand-knitted sweaters.

"Mei, look at me," Mama said. When I refused, she placed her hand on mine to stop me from pulling the loose thread of my sweatshirt. "You have to understand that there is no way to get it one hundred percent *right*, no way we can behave that will change certain people's minds about us, nowhere we can go where there won't be at least one person who will simply label us as immigrants as if that were a bad thing, or say that we're either too Chinese or too American."

Angry tears blurred my eyes as I realized she was probably right. "I'm not an immigrant," I finally said, swallowing my tears and looking at her directly, speaking with as much false confidence as I could muster. "You and Baba are. Why are you punishing me? I'm not like you."

Mama sighed, her face wearing an expression I'd seen only once before, when I'd had my first fight at the age of six. Mama had found me, inconsolable, screaming at the top of my lungs at a friend who'd inexplicably stabbed me in the leg with a pencil. I remembered sitting on Mama's lap—her rubbing my back in slow circles, her *shhh-shhh-shhh*—the stickiness of my tears, the snot I wouldn't wipe away because I wanted to show her how much I hurt. And I remembered the worry and sadness in Mama's eyes, not because of the small wound on my leg, which had already stopped bleeding, but because, I think, it was a hurt she could not explain away, a hurt that had no logic.

"I cannot make you understand." Mama stood, and pushed in her chair. "But I hope that you will try." She crossed the kitchen, removed and folded her apron and placed it inside a drawer. My tears fell, plopping on the tops of my hands as I yanked furiously on the loose thread, unraveling the hem of my sweatshirt. As I watched Mama's retreating back, my body trembled with anger, frustration. Would I ever leave the Richmond, our glass bottle, clear for everyone to see our stamped passports, question our belonging?

Every Sunday we had dinner with the first friends my parents made in the States. When the Wans, former aristocrats from Shanghai, visited us, their lively gossip with Mama and Baba filled our tiny kitchen with a jumble of Cantonese, Mandarin, Toisan, and Shanghainese. Like sparrows, my parents communicated in lyrical warbles, trilling echoes of cosmopolitan Shanghai. Our home on these nights smelled of shrimp, fermented bean paste, and green onion.

The Wans were the most adventurous people I knew: they were like the dashing bandits in the Westerns Baba and I watched together. They were the first in my parents' circle of friends to successfully digest American cheese, and Mr. Wan swam for an hour in the freezing San Francisco Bay every morning, while Mrs. Wan taught tai chi to creaky old men and women in the nearby city park. Once, they even stopped a group of bored teenagers from using bottles of bleach to poison the tide pools, shouting Chinese profanities at the tops of their lungs until the delinquents ran away. In the Wans' first year of living in San Francisco, they courageously visited nearly every neighborhood in the city, from Lake Merced to North Beach, whether they were welcome or not. The only thing they seemed to have in common with my parents was that they refused to live anywhere but the Richmond.

Mr. Wan loved to tell the story of an elderly acquaintance of his—a typewriter salesman, originally from Beijing, who traveled to downtown every morning to sell his wares. "His first day, he slipped on a step and broke his ankle, and *still* managed to sell his best typewriter before going to the hospital." Baba always shook his head in appreciation when Mr. Wan said this. "He has a limp to this day. I always ask him when he'll move in with his daughter in Sacramento, into the backyard cottage she built for him. Avocados. Oranges for miles. All sun. No more fog. No more cold, achy mornings. Make his life easier. But you know what he said?" Mr. Wan looked proudly around the table. "He said, 'I left everything once before. I'd rather break my neck than leave the Richmond.'"

Mama and Baba nodded and murmured in admiration.

While we slurped our fish-ball soup, Mrs. Wan spoke of wind in the Mission District—so strong it straightened her curls. She ran her fingers through her hair and described walking past restaurants and open kitchen windows, intoxicating aromas that were sometimes full of cumin and oregano and cinnamon. She described the diverse languages in the Mission—falling and rising tones, lively punctuated syllables, their power and musicality. She described the wonder she experienced hearing a new language for the first time. "You let the sounds wash over you like waves," she said, "and if you do not know how to swim, you trust that the deep waters will hold you. Be fearless."

"What is fearless to you?" asked Mama.

"Fearless is when you cannot understand what's being said to or around you. Fearless is celebrating, honoring, the *not* knowing. Fearless is knowing that there are histories so deep that no matter how hard you listen, you could not possibly translate all that another's heritage carries." Mrs. Wan tried to describe the familiar feeling of being surrounded by the intermingling of the old and the new, the lived-in and newly arrived. My mouth watered as she described the sweet, sugary smells wafting out the doorways of Mexican and Nicaraguan and El Salvadoran bakeries, the pastries in brilliant colors and shapes she'd never seen before.

Years later, Mama would describe fearlessness in another way. "Kinship," she said one night after dinner, years after Baba had died, as we sat back in our chairs with our full bellies, cleaning our teeth with toothpicks. "A community formed out of a need to nourish tongues with the sounds and tastes of home."

But back in 1970, on the night of my last day of sixth grade, Baba was still very much alive, and he had filled his body with whiskey and let his memories of China kick and thrash to the surface: "We here know what we left, what we lost when we escaped." He was speaking to the Wans and Mama. "People who don't *know* say that we *left* China. We didn't *leave*. It's not like a shop closing, business hours are over. No. We fled. We hid. We ran. We saw the worst in humans." The adults looked knowingly at one another. Mama nodded sadly as Baba continued. "And then . . . we found the Richmond. We persevered until white people took down the signs in their windows that read No Chinese Allowed. We carved and scraped and scoured out a *life* here." He took a gulp of whiskey, smacked his lips with satisfaction. "My wife tells me Mei wants to move out of the Richmond." Baba jabbed his thumb in my direction, then winked at Mr. Wan and Mama.

"Well, Mei, where would you go?" asked Mrs. Wan in her elegant, accented English. "What are you looking for out there?"

Trying to avoid her gaze, I glanced at Mama, then Baba; both waited for my answer with expressions I couldn't read. I shredded my napkin into my lap as I thought about leaving the Richmond to attend a swanky summer program with all the cleverest kids in my school. I imagined taking the cable car, passing underneath the deluxe skyscrapers downtown. I imagined the wind whipping through my hair in the Mission, embarking on a fearless, cumin-spiced journey into my brand-name future. I could become someone different, better, free of the Richmond's oppressive fog, its heavy white sky, the squat, unadorned buildings weighed down by their own neediness.

Finally, I spoke. "I just don't get it. What's so good about here? There's nothing. Just oily noodles and gossiping in Chinese, and a stupid school with stupid kids, and . . . what?"

Baba pushed the cork back into the whiskey bottle and said, "Belonging."

"But the Richmond isn't *ours*."

"We will keep trying to make it something of ours," Baba replied.

"But why? Why did you even come here?" My face blazed under the bright kitchen lights and glare of the adults' attentiveness. I did not yet truly understand what dangers they'd escaped, the courage it took to face the unknown. How do you teach a child about flight when that child had never heard government rifles firing into the heads of neighbors, friends, classmates; had never met the beggar poet on the street corner who shared his daily earnings with neighborhood children? I didn't know any of this as I watched Baba uncork the bottle again, pour whiskey for himself and the Wans.

At first there was nothing but the sound of the blood pounding in my ears. After a short while, Mr. Wan returned to eating. Mrs. Wan turned her attention back to my parents and started a story about her hairdresser, who had five husbands living in different parts of the city. Baba sighed, and Mama squeezed my hand under the table. After a beat, she picked up her chopsticks and popped a fish ball into her mouth while she nodded at Mrs. Wan's juicy gossip.

In the distance, I could hear the bellow of the foghorn signaling the icy low clouds rolling in off the ocean. Mama had given me a book about foghorns for my tenth birthday. On the glossy hard cover was a photo of a mammoth orange-red horn, the size of a compact car, situated below the Golden Gate Bridge's South Tower. The book said that in the 1930s, the booming foghorns used to keep residents in the Richmond awake. The city responded to the complaints by redirecting the foghorns toward the center of the Bay. I thought about the disturbed sleep of the inmates at Alcatraz, how their complaints went ignored, how the deep organ tones continued to rattle their bones until the prison was closed nearly three decades later.

The morning after the dinner party, Mama and Baba took me to the beach. We bundled up in our heaviest coats, stuffed our wool-socked feet into our shoes, and walked the three blocks to the ocean. As we sat before the choppy waves, burying our hands in the sand to warm them, we watched seagulls bob in the water and kids slap each other with long strips of seaweed.

I worked at digging a deep hole in the sand to bury a beached jellyfish. I dug diligently, occasionally looking up to watch the clouds of seafoam splatter a group of small children's ankles as they chased one another. By the time I'd finished digging, my fingers were numb and starting to prune from the dampness of the sand. I used a stick to prod the jellyfish, watched the gelatinous membrane dimple under the pressure, then tipped it into the bottom of the hole, where it wobbled briefly. I imagined myself the size of a small clam, jumping down to the bottom of this mighty hole with the jellyfish. I imagined looking up for the sun, the jellyfish waking up, thrashing against my ankles, stinging me, stinging itself until both our skins blistered and bled. I thought of how my parents' world was like the jellyfish: waterlogged, thrashing against itself— the wild translucent beauty obscured by history books; words and song and history that smelled of whiskey, of gunpowder, that presaged flight. A message for only those who knew.

I dropped down beside Mama, exhausted from digging. I plunged my fingers in the dry sand near the surface, where it had been warmed by the sun. Mama did the same. Her fingertips met mine. She smiled at me, and after a moment said, "Remember that report you did about the dodo?"

I nodded.

"You were so upset about that silly bird, about how they all died out, got themselves killed by humans." As she used her other hand to pile sand on top of our buried ones, I thought about how I'd asked Mama over and over why the universe had doomed these heavy-beaked, feathery reptiles to extinction. Had created them, but given them no way to defend themselves. For the report, instead of drawing pictures of the dodo, I drew pictures of Mama sucking in her breath, then holding it. She held in so much air that red dots bloomed on her puffed cheeks. The air lifted her off the ground and into the air. Did birds do the same thing in order to fly?

One of the children near us on the beach was being picked on by some teenagers. The child threw her bucket at them, but the wind grabbed it and splashed it into the water. Unable to reach the pail without wading into the frigid tide, she cried in frustration. Mama looked on, a proud smile on her face, as Baba stood and wiped sand off his butt, then jogged down to the water to retrieve the bucket.

"We left our home to make our new life, Mei," she said. "And it was here we had you. Here we met the Wans. Here we made do the best we could. You weren't there when we fled our homes with nothing but what we could sew into the linings of our jackets. My whole life was running, Mei. Your father and I, we are done searching. We belong here. Do you understand?"

I wanted to say that I did. I wanted to say that I understood hunger, that I understood why China's farmers would slaughter the country's sparrows, and why in 1958 this meant that locusts leapt from the clouds instead of rain. I wanted to say that I understood why Mama cried when she told stories of this plague, this famine, collectivized starvation. I wanted to say that I understood Baba's crude jokes with the Wans, about how they'd escaped genocide by pointing to their neighbors then playing dead. But at eleven, I couldn't interpret their birdsong and thought it a sweet uselessness. I couldn't grasp my parents' twisted refugee humor or that their laughter was a sparrow song of sorrow, of disloyalty, of survival—a savage happiness. I couldn't picture Mama's childhood friend on her knees, hands tied behind her back, hair spilling over her shoulders, tears pouring from her eyes as a soldier towered over her. I could not picture the explosion of a bullet fired from a rifle, the pierced skin, the shattering skull, the blood, or Mama's grief. That knowledge, those images, would come later. But at eleven, I had not lost something, anything, anyone, so dear, never witnessed such violence.

Mama exhaled, squeezed my hand again under the sand, then stood. She brushed off her legs and trotted down to join Baba by the water.

From where I sat high up on the beach, my back snug against the dunes, Baba and Mama looked like little miniatures of themselves. Baba's sunglasses just a black strip around his head, like a little bandit mask. I pictured my parents as little figurines molded out of wet sand, clutching the pail's curved lip as they bobbed in the water, traveling thousands of miles from home, looking up into to a new skyline in the distance, full of towering telephone poles, electric lines, fog.

MOM'S DESERT

1

Smell of slick summer fog and wet asphalt. San Francisco. 1966. On Mom's first date with my father, she agreed to "copilot" his motorcycle. She wore sandals and a flowing magenta skirt hitched up and knotted at her thighs. When they crashed, Mom was thrown onto a grassy median, but not before the concrete curb tore off her toenails. My father, unluckier, slid across the road, shredding half of his leg skin. Still, he carried Mom in his arms up the steps of a blue house, placed her gently down, then passed out. Mom lay there on the porch, bleeding with him, her pulpy toes soft as squash soup.

They shared a room in the hospital. When I imagine this scene, I see their four legs hitched in the air. For weeks, they shared the same pus-and-bandaged-sweat smells. That sort of rubbery, meaty, salty odor you can't get enough of, especially when it's your own, or that of someone you love. They had more doctor's dates, full of limping and scab-picking and ointment. Then, they had me.

2

Mom cooked breakfast for dinner: flat fried eggs propped up on torn chunks of buttered baguette. I was eight. Mom sipped wine and watched me watching her toes; her big right toenail was still missing. Nine nails had grown back: thick, opaque, and without the faint white crescents below the cuticles. I imagined the original ten, painted magenta to match Mom's skirt, scattered and buried in the grassy median. In their place grew neon pink earthworms, bright fuchsia pebbles, coral gophers.

Dad was an amateur actor and a holiday music freak deeply in love with steak sauce. Mom was talking about him on the phone to her friend while I ate. She was describing how she'd caught Dad the previous week squeezing a young actress's "peaches" in his dressing room at the community theater. "I just screamed SEX! from the doorway. I didn't know what else to do." She reported with sad satisfaction that Dad had frantically stuffed his excited "grapes" back in his jeans, snagging skin in the zipper, that he'd howled.

"Why did he do it?" I asked when she hung up.

Mom did not answer my question; instead, blocked the salt shaker with her paw when I tried to use it on my eggs. "Too much," she said, rigid and pointed as my fork.

I pushed my plate away.

"Why don't you finish your food? Do you think eggs grow on trees?" She dug into imaginary empty pockets and commanded her lap: "Money, come out!"

I smiled despite myself.

"Why are you smiling?"

"Because you are."

"No. You misread my face."

I kept quiet, sat on my real thoughts like a bird warming its eggs high up in a tree. I thought of how, when the time was right, when the excitement was near, I would get up and just let those eggs roll out the nest. Crash! Splat! Tender, yellow and wet.

3

Mom was raised on the hot arid western edge of China. She often juxtaposed our foggy ocean beach to the blazing sands and flash floods of her youth. She described the idiots riding waves on plywood, the rising water's roar, her family's poverty, and her rural desert upbringing. She once told my father that she'll know she's made it in life when she has a fridge with an icemaker.

After Dad left us, we moved to a new apartment with a view of Lake Merritt and an icemaker. Mom left our ice cube trays in our old freezer, stacked, empty, ready for someone else's cold, clear water.

4

The horoscope for Pisces in the Sunday *Chronicle* read, "Water is life. But true love is smell. If you love someone's smell, it's true love."

"Then you must true love Beatrice." Mom poked me playfully with her big toe. She was thinking of how I liked to run my fingers along the inside of our twelve-year-old bulldog's drooping lips, then smell the wetness. It was all mossy and meaty and decaying wood. And when Beatrice yawned, I stuck my face right *inside* her gentle underbite.

The day Dad moved out, Mom let him bury his nose in her long black hair, still damp from her morning shower and smelling of citrus and rose; he told her that he loved her shampoo.

I think, now, that this was him saying sorry.

I remember these things about that day, too:

Going to the beach so we wouldn't have to watch Dad pack his things.

The foghorn's slow deep bellow.

Finding a stranded baby sea turtle, its enormous shell heavy, round and brown as our coffee table.

Black sand fleas swarming our ankles and the turtle's leathery flippers.

Beatrice licking the turtle's large black eye.

The long track carved in the sand where the turtle had dragged itself from the water.

Begging Mom to drive the turtle to the animal hospital.

Mom sounding like a disapproving scientist when she said, "The turtle should die on this beach. It shouldn't die in the back of a Subaru."

Mom watching me watch the turtle.

5

On our way home from the emergency animal clinic, we were pulled over for making a wrong turn down a one-way street. It was a cold evening. My ankles itched, blooming with cherry-red spots, first-rate beach rash. I pushed my nose into Beatrice's face folds, smelled a million things at once: ocean saltiness, seaweed, dead turtle, sweet and putrid. When the policeman returned to his patrol car, Mom smacked the steering wheel with her palm, whispered fiercely, "This cop's an asshole! That vet was an asshole!" The veterinarian had lectured Mom on the importance of leaving wildlife in its natural habitat, especially a turtle that was already dead. Mom had nodded obediently, fists clenched below the counter, her long nails digging deep red crescents in her palms. I did the same, in solidarity, as if to say, "It's not our fault," though my nails were too short to leave any markings.

Mom checked her rearview mirror, frowned at the cop writing our ticket. There was a sound down the street; someone shouting a woman's name. Maybe for their cat? Maybe their mom? The night clouds hung low, dark and cool.

Mom said, "I just feel like . . . I just want to turn right, and the whole world is turning left."

I nodded, watched the light from passing cars illuminate the brown age spot on Mom's cheek and the sunburned tops of my knees, and I thought, *Shiny us*. Beatrice crawled over the armrest onto my lap, and I scratched her belly, released the deepest scent of her fur into the air. Biscuits and toasted bread. My fingers traced the tiny brown scar on her stomach where she once had her puppy belly torn by the vet, insides shifted—no more room for puppies. I thought: *Fingers and skin remember*. Beatrice barked. I made a ring with my hands and muzzled her snout; she pulled away, but I held tight.

After I let go, I asked Mom, "Why didn't you want to save the turtle?"

"I don't know." She shook her head. "Why did *you*?"

6

After school, in our new kitchen, I watched Mom fill a glass with ice for my apple juice. I held up a piece of paper marked up with bright red slashes and a big letter C circled three times at the top. I proclaimed, "Math is an asshole!" Mom's laughter, sad and generous, sounded like a flash flood moving at top speed. I pictured Mom's desert, the parched grasses bleached white by a white sun, the winds picking up, silvery clouds rolling in. I pictured myself scrambling on the sandy dunes toward the waves. Cheering wantonly though glued to the shore. Mom's toes digging into the wet sand—spoons in pudding. I pictured the fervor and risk, the overheated dreams of those idiots on plywood. And Mom, waiting to cross all night; she would wait, *unglued*, edging closer to the crumbling shore as the world rushed by.

THE FOX SPIRIT

Elder Sister had a river-rock forehead, perfectly rounded and sleek. She had pointed ears like a fox. The women in our mountain village were skilled seamstresses and made their own clothes, but Elder Sister outshone them all. Her black robes were adorned with the brightest reds and greens. From small tin squares she cut strips like tendrils, then embroidered her favorite spirits, the fox and beetle, into thick wooly fabric with the silvery thread. We were not wealthy, but she wore silver necklaces even when it was not Spring Festival. She told me that as the elder daughter of the village priest, she must maintain *face*, to show the villagers how Father had raised a dignified family outside of the temple. Mother and Father barely looked at me when she and I were in the same room. You could not blame them. Elder Sister shone so brightly.

I was always an avid storyteller, but I was especially dedicated in those winter months during Elder Sister's fever. My stories were intended to fill her dreams with color and animals and magic. I wanted bright orange tigers bounding in and out of the jungles of her mind, and hoary goats scaling the tallest peaks so that their heads jutted through the clouds. Sometimes the dreams stirred her; she giggled, her teeth chattered, and she cursed foully. Mother clucked her tongue, displeased at the dirty language, and I marveled at how she sounded like a woodpecker. She even looked like one when her ashy hair was wound into a tight bun, and when her beady eyes darted around Elder Sister's room, looking for places where the illness might hide. Her sharp eyes glowed yellow, reflecting the dim bedside candle that she kept burning day and night. Mother's anxious bird sounds, the perpetual winter darkness, and the cursing all intensified as Elder Sister's fever burned.

Kneeling at the edge of Elder Sister's bed, I noted how her throat burbled like a dying fish while she slept. I whispered into her ear, *I need you. Please listen to my story.* I held her hand, but her fingers rested limply in mine. I thought of the nights she had played pipa, lively music to accompany my stories. I thought of the strummed beat in the air, of her strong hands on those strings, how her sounds deepened my imagination. I thought of my fictional heroines triumphing over the ogres, the ruin, blood, and madness they battled. At her bedside, I exercised Elder Sister's fingers, slowly flexed each one. I watched for her expression to change, but there was no struggle in her face, no war or campaign.

Mother entered with a pot of steaming tea, placed it on the bedside table, and tiredly sat down beside me. I studied her lips, her cheeks, thought of how they were once so full and red. The best of our vegetables and dried meats went into medicinal soups for Elder Sister. My stomach, empty and twisted, grumbled and complained.

Before Elder Sister's illness, I'd fill my stories with characters eating large red apples, breaking the skin with their teeth, letting the juice run down their chins. In my tales our family grew fat on flour-battered fried fish, succulent roasted pigs dripping in peanut oil, egg custard tarts with sunny yellow centers and golden crusts.

A feast, she would always say. *More than we could ever need.*

In my hungriest hours, I resented Elder Sister. I thought of how she must have savored my stories, stockpiled her dreams with our family's food. I wondered how many more months our family could survive with our meager pantry and my waning imagination.

Mother tried to wrap her sweater tighter around her shoulders. Our elbows knocked.

"You take up too much space."

"No, I don't." I admired the hand-rubbed quilt fabric, dyed in indigo, deep blue like water. Mother tucked the edges of it under the thin mattress, kneaded the blood and warmth back into my sister's fingers. Elder Sister's arms were sleeved in heavily wrinkled brown cotton, like the rough bark of a tree. When I blurred my eyes, it looked as if Mother were massaging her branches. "Let me stay," I begged.

Mother sighed—her breath smelled of ashes—then shooed me from the room.

I left to wander along the cold river, alone. From the banks, I felt a heavy pull on my limbs; rocks filled my stomach. To keep myself company, I cursed aloud at Mother, the dark, the cold—at all the wickedness that kept me from Elder Sister.

From the silty shallows of the river, two foxes suddenly formed. At first, I pretended to ignore them; I didn't have anything to feed them and thought they would be scared if I reached out. I stayed perfectly still, like a statue. I admired their slicked fur, silver in the moonlight, a hardened shell of clay. The foxes circled me for several minutes, eyeing me warily. One finally approached, sniffed the air around my mouth, its nose a glossy black river stone. I extended my hand to stroke its fur, and to my great surprise, the fox spoke.

Elder Sister is sinking in dark waters, the fox whispered, its icy breath ghosting my ear.

Without sunlight, your sister's mind is flat and still, said the other fox as it nibbled on some nearby moss.

How do I find a way into her dreams? How do I save her? I asked.

The foxes shook out their fur, spattering my clothes with flecks of mud. They stretched, chins up, rear legs extended backward, their claws scraping the dirt ground. They sighed as if bored by my questions. *Isn't it obvious?* said one fox as it licked its paw. *You must warm her.*

I plucked some grass and held it out to the foxes, who nibbled the frostbitten green blades, smacked their lips, blinked sleepily. *Fire-eating beetles will help you if you feed them. Find the beetles. Their blazing tongues can push the sun into the sky, and morning will come, and you will warm your sister.* They twitched their pointed ears; moonlight glinted off their eyes. *Without Elder Sister, you will have no stories to tell. No one to listen.*

My breath caught. *If Elder Sister dies . . .*

The foxes suddenly began to shiver violently, their bodies cracking. I leapt up and scooped up the shards of mud falling from their fur, tried to mix them with handfuls of water to soften them, tried but could not reattach them. I was terrified of what would happen when the foxes became fully unshelled.

Please, don't go, I pleaded. *Please. I am too little. Insignificant. I cannot do it alone.*

Is that how you want to be? Invisible? To think yourself so small that you eat only in little hard bites? Why would you carry a letter instead of deliver it? they asked with their final fading breaths.

Their question was not posed out of scorn. It was an acknowledgment of the hunger of an invisible child. It was giving that child fistfuls of steaming rice. It was showing how potatoes send out new roots even after they've been ripped from the earth. It was teaching how to eat the whole lemon, biting into the skin, admiring the teethmarks in the yellow flesh while chewing and licking the sour.

I want to be seen, I said minutes later, to the pile of mud that soon lay at my feet. *I will not stay hidden.*

Father kept a library for his priest papers and cloth scrolls—a small room adjoining the kitchen that I was forbidden from entering. But I was no longer afraid. The foxes had shown me the path, the healing power of the scrolls, the power I needed to make my own. After I returned home, I slid the doorway's heavy wool curtains aside and stepped into the library. I held my breath, letting the panels fall back into place. While the house slumbered, I pulled papers from wooden cases, spread everything out on the ground, and drew over the sacred symbols with a charcoal stick. I drew Elder Sister's silk dress, made heavy with her embroidery of foxes and beetles—luminous silver chains wound tight around her neck. I drew Father in his priest robes and riding atop a shadow dog. I drew Mother on a galloping horse carved of honey locust soap, splashing through puddles of lather. In my pictures, Elder Sister rode on her own horse alongside Father and my sudsy mother, her flapping, wrinkled sleeves grazing evergreen firs as she flew by, knocking snow from the fine-toothed needles. In my pictures, I led the way, shouting instructions to everyone for where to go. My fingers tingled with so much magic I could barely hold the horse's reigns through its icy gallop, each foggy breath a thrill.

In the deepest part of the night, a man pounded on our front door, begging to be let in. Father pulled on his thick winter robes, instinctively knowing that a call at this hour would be for him, a call that meant a family might have lost someone to the same sickness that plagued Elder Sister. I hid my charcoal-blackened hands in my sleep-robe's pockets. "You should accompany me, learn how I bury ghosts," Father said, even though he knew I never touched the dead. I followed him to the door, stood in front of the curtain to Father's library. I shook my head guiltily and looked down at my toes; I was ashamed at my relief that Father would not go into his library that morning and see my drawings, that the other family's suffering meant my secret efforts would remain hidden until I was ready.

As soon as Father departed, the memory of the silver foxes nipped at my legs. It was time. *Now. Hurry*, they said. I bounded out of the house with my drawings and Father's sacred cloth scrolls stuffed inside my robes. My eyes scanned left, then right, to make certain that Father had gone. I cut through the cinnamon forest that surrounded our house, scuttling low to the ground, occasionally crouching into a squat to survey the path to the temple. Would Elder Sister laugh if she saw how I teetered like an unstable shore crab? I headed north toward the river and prayed that in crossing the bridge, which was brightly lit by the full moon, I would not be caught.

I counted my steps as I picked my way up the temple's stone pathway. Once inside, I placed my heavy bundle at the feet of the wooden statue of a cloaked woman cradling an egret, Father's favorite goddess. I jammed a burning incense stick into the center of my holy shrine, fell to my knees, and prayed that the silver foxes were right, that fire-eating beetles would steal Elder Sister's fever from her.

The fire grew slowly, and I watched them from up close. When the beetles appeared at last, smoke poured from their tiny nostrils as they danced in the scented flames. I got up and threw my arms wide, twirled and stomped my feet. I shrieked in jubilant anger, filled the grand temple with my resentment. In the smoke, my loneliness and invisibility found their home. Soon the floor began to vibrate, the walls shook as if made of twigs. Jagged flames leapt up toward the temple spire, a signal beacon, and the goddess crumpled to her knees; I gasped with delight as her necklace of fire shone even more brightly than Elder Sister's silver chains. I stayed until the roar became too much and the great heat pushed me outside.

When the villagers came with their buckets of water from the nearby creek, they did not see me, covered in soot, crouched in the shadow of a tree. Father, fully dressed in his priest robes, was the first of my family to arrive. From my hiding place, I watched him start toward the line of those passing buckets back and forth, then stop abruptly midstride. I wondered if he had, for one guilty moment, considered how he could fight the fire without ruining his elegant robes.

Mother arrived soon after, and my breath caught when I saw she brought Elder Sister, whose forehead glistened, pale with sweat, as she stepped carefully, as if she did not trust her legs to keep her up. I watched the field of shimmering grief-stricken faces. I watched Mother, her eyes bright, mouth open. And I watched Father cradle his head in his soot-black hands. And yet I felt powerful. It was I who had fed the fire-eating beetles, I who had made morning come, and it was I who stirred my sister from her feeble dreams. Elder Sister leaned on Mother for support, and I wondered if she knew what I had done for her. I wondered if she had looked over at my empty bed when Mother shook her awake, whether she worried because I was not there. I wondered if Mother remembered me at all.

When the beetles had tired of feeding, they hurled the sun into the sky, where it perched unsteadily atop Mount Luohan, burning, burning. I briefly lost my hiding place in the shadows, but when the winter frost met the fire's heat, a rancid fog grew and I was obscured once more. Villagers, one by one, dropped out of the fight to save our temple, no longer able to work in the stifling haze. I trembled with anticipation as I waited for the fog to clear so that my weary audience would turn their attention to me.

Father, Mother, and Elder Sister had not moved since they arrived. But when one elderly woman stumbled in front of them and splashed water all over, Mother helped her up, set her safely beside a tree, then took up the bucket and set out for the creek to retrieve more water. Father looked like he would be sick as he watched his wife struggle with the heavy bucket, her legs coated in mud. He tried to brush the splatters and soot from his robes, but even from where I stood, I could see that the fabric was hopelessly stained. With a deep breath, he stripped down to his linen pants and undershirt, waded into the water up to his waist. The villagers, heartbroken to see their spiritual leader filling buckets, reformed their line and worked diligently alongside Father and Mother to douse the fire. Elder Sister stood perfectly still, her gaze haunted, as if she believed she had not woken up and was inside of a nightmare. She began shivering, though she was just feet from the flames.

The silver foxes nudged me forward. I walked out from the shelter of the cinnamon tree and, for the first time since the fire started, stood straight. I lifted my arms to the heavens, and in my powerful storyteller voice, I praised the silver foxes and fire-eating beetles.

"Thank you," I said. "You helped me bring the sun, and now I have healed my sister."

The villagers circled around me to listen, and some dropped to their knees to weep at my words. I felt their sorrow, more bitter than the smoke. A breeze blew the acrid haze across the wet field; my eyes and nose stung. I turned and looked expectantly at my family. *Look at me*, I begged silently. I wanted them to see how powerful I had become. *Please, please, look at me*. But they remained motionless, their faces contorted as they watched the burning temple.

I walked over and clutched Elder Sister's trembling hand. I looked up at her, pleadingly. At first she did nothing, and we also watched the smoldering embers of the temple, of Father's goddess, of our village's most sacred place. But after a while, she squeezed my hand, and I felt it in my heart. The curved stone path that had led me to the temple's entrance was also destroyed; small rock islands jutted out of a river of ash. The cloaked goddess was nothing more than a blackened stump at our feet. My drawings, of course, had been devoured by the voracious beetle spirits, and I knew that I would never find them. The temple's carved wooden spire, which had once reached as high as the treetops, was gone. I looked up at the blue-black wound in the sky where it used to be and realized that I could not remember exactly what it looked like. I could not remember what animal spirits our ancestors had carved into the wood, whether they had included the fox spirit or fire-eating beetles. I closed my eyes and saw my sister's face, and for the first time considered how the cool darkness may have comforted her when her fever raged. I saw the flicker of Mother's candles. And I saw my father, again in his splendid robes, sweeping from the house to quell the stormy grief of the parents of a dead child. And finally, I felt my own grief rise.

Elder Sister leaned into my ear and spoke in a hoarse whisper, her throat constricted by the smoke; I could not hear what she said, but I imagined it: *I can hear you, Little Sister. I know your struggle.* My eyes blurred, and I closed them so that I could not see how the villagers looked at me—so I could not see how Father and Mother would not.

SPIDER LOVE SONG

The fisherwoman lays down her box of tackle, drops a tattered yellow beach chair from her shoulder, jams her fishing rod into the sand, line and red plastic ball swinging in the wind. From the window of the cottage, ten-year-old Sophie Chu studies the woman's short gray coat, jeans, spindly legs tucked into tall rubber boots, skin the color of wet sand, and black hair with streaks of ash.

"Time for lunch?" asks Sophie.

Sophie's grandmother, hard of hearing over the crush of waves, asks in Cantonese, "Repeat?"

It is almost noon. Sophie's empty stomach churns on itself; her frozen earlobes peek from under her sweatband; her paper elephant ears flap in the wind. Sophie rests her cheek on Grandmother's stomach to warm it. The stomach growls.

Posters of Sophie's missing parents were plastered all around the small coastal village, affixed to powerline poles along the narrow dusty roads, tacked to hay bales in the busiest pastures full of sweet brown cows, the fliers pierced by baling wire in neighboring cornfields. Sophie had used their wedding photo, where the newlyweds posed on a misty ocean bluff, looking over their shoulders at the camera, grinning as if they were running away. Her mother's hair, a tangle blowing in the wind. Their sepia-toned smiles bright as cantaloupe slices. Sophie included a description of the car they'd been driving.

Over the months since they'd vanished, their smiling faces had been scrawled with mustaches and eye patches and blackened teeth gaps and lion-mane ruffs and hog ears. And before long, other posters covered her parents' faces, thumbtacks speared through their paper foreheads: a lost narcoleptic curly-haired dog, a water-logged piano that needed a new home, an emaciated and milkless goat for sale, a senile grandfather who was obsessed with seaweed.

Sophie often thinks of the morning her parents went missing, how she cradled the large box of doughnuts, standing in the bakery with Grandmother—smears of rich coconut filling, pineapple sugar-crusted buns, deep red bean paste—her eight-year-old heart thumping a steady beat, anxious to bring the sweetness home to her tired parents, whom she thought were asleep in their bed. She remembers how Grandmother bragged to the other patrons until the silky oil blooms on the bottom of the box saturated Sophie's fuzzy elephant arms so that she smelled like a doughnut, how Sophie carried that scent home, how she still smelled hours later when Grandmother called the neighbors and then the village hospital in search of her missing daughter and son-in-law. How, as Sophie fell sleep on the couch listening to the uneasy drone of Grandmother on the phone with relatives, she buried her nose deep in her elephant arms, trying to pull clues from the downy fibers.

The fisherwoman knocks on their bright red cottage door, asks to use their phone to call a tow truck.

It will be a forty-minute wait.

Sophie and Grandmother learn that the woman's name is Gail "Owl" Yip. Owl does not know why Owl. It was a name she was given in college, she says—the same one Sophie's parents had attended, back in the city, where Owl had become a journalist. The woman goes on to describe the room that she and Sophie's mother once shared as young students, the long walks home from the college to their cramped apartment each evening.

Sophie, who had heard every story told by her parents about the days when they met in school, knows that her mother had lived at home and made the long tiring drive in to the college each day. She has never heard of Owl. Sophie determines the woman has never actually known Sophie's parents. She is there to snoop. But Sophie does not have the heart to tell Grandmother, who, once so sociable, no longer lets strangers visit, who detests the town gossip and the stories the neighbors tell one another as they sip coffee and speculate about what happened to her parents.

Owl surveys the small cottage, sits on one of the two matching brown chairs in the cramped living room, studies the deep navy walls, the cracked paint, the stains on her armrests, the rough walnut floors. She tells Sophie that she remembered her dear old friends had had a daughter, but didn't know they'd named her Sophie. "What a lovely name," she says.

Sophie shivers as she warms her hands over the radiator; the only people she and Grandmother have allowed in their home since her parents' disappearance are the sheriff, the podiatrist who clips Grandmother's toenails and checks her blood pressure, and Grandmother's quilting club, which consists of five elderly women who never speak.

Owl picks up two hard-covered books written in Braille. "What's this one?"

Sophie squints in the dimness, recognizes the orange and red covers. "That one? *On Napoleon and Night Writing.*"

"And the other?"

"*Braille: Six Dots to Success.*"

"What are they about?" asks Owl.

"How Napoleon used too many dots in his army code so no one, not even his own army, could figure it out."

"How many dots?" asks Owl.

"Twelve."

"And the other book?"

"Mr. Braille figured how to do it in six."

Owl nods admiringly, studies the long spines of the books, flips through the thick white pages, runs her fingertips along the raised dots. Where there would be color photos of Napoleon—his pointed nose and hat—there were instead embossed outlines of his portrait. Sophie watches as the woman places her entire hand over the famous general's face, as if feeling for fever, and then pushes her nose into the open book and inhales deeply.

"Why do you need these?" Owl asks Grandmother. "You're not blind. Are you?" Owl squats in front of Grandmother, waves her arms slowly in the old woman's line of sight. Grandmother flicks the air in front of her face, as if swatting a bird that just fell from the sky, heavy, like a stone.

Sophie Chu's Journal: I am a cat. I am hiding in the closet. There is a window, and I know that it is almost time for me to cook. I am seated on top of the piles of clothes. They are wrapped in plastic like dead bodies. My knees are pulled up to my chest. It is nighttime but I wish that it was daytime because my window lets in the light and warms the tiny closet, makes it feel like a real room. When I hide here, Grandmother always finds me, and I always ask, "How did you know?" And she always says, "Where else would you be?"

Finding is not always bad. I am not a very good swimmer, but if I have to I can splash and kick my legs wildly until I am moving somewhere. I am a loud swimmer, that's what Grandmother says. She likes that because she can always find me in a crowded pool.

I am not stretched plastic. I am bunched up, and it feels good sometimes to squeeze into the tiniest spaces to remind myself of how big I've gotten. I am growing at the speed of light.

I am facing the closet door, which is closed because that's better for hiding. On my left there are more bags of clothes. On my right there is the window, small, high up. I have to stand on the bags to see outside. Outside there is a small patch of concrete that Father poured, and a basketball hoop. I am good at basketball when I want to be. Behind me are more bags of clothes. None of the clothes are mine.

I am certain there is going to be an earthquake one day and the bags will come tumbling out of the closet like an avalanche. The door doesn't close properly, it is crooked and heavy, and the paint is nice and thick, so it just sort of sticks shut. I like that. I like when things don't work, but they do.

Sophie goes to the kitchen, tries to eavesdrop over the sound of oil bubbling in the wok; under the rich gurgling notes, she hears just chipped murmurs of Grandmother and Owl. Outside the window is her mother's planter box filled with yolky buttercups, milky daisies, iridescent violet snapdragons, and the low tremolo whirring of a small black bird with a rosy throat and a rich brown head.

Sophie carries in a tray to the two women: green tea served in small ceramic bowls and steaming caramel-colored blocks of fried soybean cakes soaked in soy sauce. Sophie sucks on a soybean cube, squeezes it into a salty pulp between her cheek and her teeth, uses her tongue to masticate it against the roof of her mouth. Grandmother slurps her tea approvingly. Highest compliment.

Owl plucks a tofu cube, nibbles a corner of it before putting it down on the edge of her tea plate, continues her perusal of one of the books, the bumpy white pages like two white frog bellies, opened, curved, held in place by her thumbs. She pauses to run her hands along the pages of a book about trains, and again for a book about ducks. She asks, "So, your parents. Have you heard from them?" She cranes her neck toward the dark hallway leading to the bedrooms, as though expecting two grown-ups to suddenly peek their heads out.

Grandmother opens her mouth and swiftly leans in as if to speak, but instead lets out a series of low burps, *chup-chup-chuuup,* and then sits back and smiles at the room; Sophie is reminded of the sound of warblers hunting, tiny but fearless, adept in the air, catching flying insects on the wing.

"People in town say that you have quite a special gift for cooking," says Owl. "Did your mother teach you?"

Grandmother pops an entire tofu cube in her mouth. She tosses in another and another before she starts chewing. "I want to remember every good taste," the old woman says, mouth full. "Do we remember tastes the same way we remember smells? I'm surrounded by everything good here." She pats Sophie's hand, goes on to describe how her own father had entered a radio jingle contest because the first prize was a powerful electric hand drill, but he won second place, a goldfish in a bag, which doesn't really help someone who needs a hand drill.

Sophie thinks of the meal that she has planned for tonight: two splendid frogs wrapped in butcher paper and sprinkled with finely powdered sawdust to keep the skin from sticking, ripping. She had placed them in the crisper, frogs so fresh they were just that morning hopping and clinging to the edges of the village fishmonger's portable aquarium (aka bucket). After Owl leaves, Sophie will wash the frogs under the faucet, water cold enough to make her skin goose-pimple, her arm hairs stand in salute. The clean froggy flesh will be wet, shining, mottled green and white and brown. Blue-tinged blotches and dots. She will lay them out on the counter, run a long silver knife along their bellies, and watch the red line bloom beneath the skins, the intestines spilling out like thick wet yarn. Grandmother will help with simpler tasks, scooping out the silky organs, placing them in a coffee mug.

Recipe for tender frog skin from an ancient book she'd found in the attic:

Soak
flesh
wash
rinse

drum
beat
stretch
oil
drum
beat

They will broil the frog thighs in the oven—pearlescent moon slivers—with pungent garlic, tiny onions, then serve them on a bed of peppery baby arugula. They will chew the meat, and later, make loud croaking burps.

"You must be a pretty smart elephant to figure out this Braille stuff," says Owl. "Your parents must be so proud of you."

Grandmother's ears perk up; she tilts her head, wears a solemn expression as if she'd heard something different than what Sophie heard.

Sophie shivers again; she hadn't thought that Braille or knowing how to cook frogs made her a more special elephant. She cannot always remember what her parents look like; in her mind she sees their smiling faces, sometimes with pirate eye-patches, sometimes with missing teeth, with pig ears. She sometimes forgets the difference between *melon* and *lemon*, because the letters scramble up. But she can scramble powdered eggs so they taste fresh from the shell. She can fry up sausages—oily, salty skin so crisp it shatters in your mouth like glass.

Owl drags her heels when she walks, just as Sophie's parents did after a long shift at the hospital, coming in to tell stories to Sophie, waking her up just to say goodnight. Sophie remembers those nights, her mother's breath close to her cheek as she whispered *Sweet dreams*, and how Sophie would grip her mother's wrist, pulling her back, asking about her day's adventures. She remembers how on nights with full moons, she could see her mother's face contort, pondering if she should answer. Some nights, her mother would shush Sophie and retrace her steps out of the room,

93

closing the door behind her with a firm *click*. Other nights she would brush Sophie's tangled hair with her fingers and tell her about a man brought into the hospital, wheeled in on a gurney just to be declared dead, a pile of blood and bone and skin. Everything rich red, throbbing, oyster soft. Sophie remembers how her mother's breath smelled like milk warming on the stovetop, rich with foam, the raw sourness boiled off with the steam.

Sophie watches as static from Owl's restless shifting in the chair makes the hairs at the top of Owl's head rise up, strands like a deep sea creature's tentacles waving to passing ships.

"What's this?" Owl holds out a bird's nest resembling a twiggy cup.

"Grandmother says it's a warbler's."

"This?" Owl cradles a small black rock in her hand, the size of a penny, glossy, with a graphic white spiral in the center. She moves to stand in front of the living room window; the fading afternoon light from outside silhouettes her so that she resembles someone haunted.

"A fossil."

Owl gives a low hooting whistle, eyebrows cocked.

"It's, like, four hundred fifty thousand years old and used to live under the ocean."

"A real treasure!"

"Grandma paid five dollars at the magic shop."

"You sure are a special kid to know so much."

Sophie cannot remember the last time she'd been told that something she did was special; at school she was teased constantly for her old elephant skin. At first, the kids, curious, craned their necks for better views as she strode down the hallway to class—they reached out to touch her woolly gray arms, to tug her white-and-blue striped trunk, to flick her floppy gray ears, to squeeze her long tail. They begged their parents for their own elephants, begged Sophie to teach them how to become one. She gave advice: Be bigger than life, stomp your heavy elephant feet, trust your trunk and wrap it around your cranberry juice box and *squeeze!*

But after months of elephant life, Sophie began to stink: an onion left in a hot car all day, or ground beef graying on the kitchen counter, or a hot wet sock running around in a soggy shoe.

The kinder kids, the ones with noses like bloodhounds, begged to do her laundry, offered to bring her home with them because their mommies were the *best* at getting stink out. Some kids would pinch their noses dramatically as they passed her in the cafeteria, bathroom, hallway, classroom desk. The school's regular bully—a boy with a crafty reputation, hair like a tumbleweed, who claimed to be a descendant of California's first potato king; a boy who had held his tongue during the weeks when helicopters circled the village coastline in search of the red Saab, whirring blades stirring up dust and excitement for everyone—revved up his bully engine with slurring, plaintive taunts that wrapped like ribbons around Sophie's throat:

Sophie, dummy Sophie. Seep-seep-seep! Living with crazy grandma. Chatter-chatter, bubble-bubble, rot. Did your mommy and daddy find a better life in the city or are they worms and sod? Schick-schick—dick! What happens when you take off your stupid ears, your stupid trunk? Where does your elephant go? What happens when you peel a dog?

Sophie's first costume was not of an elephant. Grandmother had stayed up with her the night before Halloween, helped her build different costumes made from clothing and utensils and odds and ends from the house. Sophie's first attempt at a costume was that of a big game hunter. She'd pulled all of the khaki-colored clothing from her parents' closets, from the attic trunk, from Grandmother's collection of sewing fabric. She'd even shaved the neighbor's cat into a lion, leaving just a tuft of fur around its face, neck, and the tip of its tail. But building a replica rifle out of cooking utensils proved too difficult. The second costume they tried was a swan,

but it would have taken more than the two pillows they'd torn apart
to get to the feathers fluffy, and the paste that Sophie used to glue
the feathers on was making her arms and legs break out in hives.
The third costume was a nightmare bat. The frame for the wings
was built out of wire hangers, extending from her body as if she
were about to take off in a flat-winged glide. But the black felted
fabric was too heavy for the hangers, and the bent wire cut into
the skin on Sophie's shoulders and scraped the floor as she walked.

"What do you most want to become?" asked Grandmother. "If
you were this *person*, really *this person*, who would you most want
to *be*?"

The elephant costume came as a lightning bolt of inspiration.
The voluminous gray coat that Sophie found in the garage was
what her father wore when he had to clear the storm drains during
hurricanes. And the tube sock was her mother's, from a pair she
had when she'd played badminton on Saturdays with the neighbors,
before Grandmother's declining health took up the bulk of her
time when home.

Elephants lived long lives; their mammoth memories could
make the grandest storyteller blush. An elephant towered over
everything, everyone, yet could curl its firehose trunk around a
branch, pluck a green leaf whole. What power! What bigness! What
sensitivity!

Sophie's parents brought home death every day, stories that
kept her up for hours some nights, stories of men with blood dripping out of their ears, men with cheekbones protruding through
their eye sockets, eyeballs skewered like soft-boiled eggs. Sophie
imagined an elephant's brain stem, how it might feel ripping
through the base of its colossal skull. On the tongue, would it be
bitter and hard like the woody stem of an apple? Would it prick
like a burr? Would it crease and snap like fresh spinach?

She'd heard stories that turned her stomach inside out, stories
of young women, girls not much older than herself, forced to bear

children before their bodies could manage that type of ripping pain. Her mother described the fistulas that formed, the gaping holes where their vaginas should be, limp meatball tunnels, openings that would not close without surgery, where their organs and shit and blood would come rushing out. Sophie remembers falling asleep, staring at her peeling ceiling, the worn wallpaper, imagining the bedroom walls tumbling down.

Sophie Chu's Journal: I am cures. I am full of them. My recipe books are packed with everything she's taught me. How to repair broken seams, to quell hunger, to temper nausea. I am full of everything.

I am a sad sack tonight. I am inside the sack. It is cotton, and there are tiny pinprick moth holes that I can see out of. I am sitting inside the sack, pressing my face against the fabric to breathe. I am there, it is nighttime, and my bed turns into a sack when I can't get to sleep because my memories are keeping me up. I am alone but my memories are there. It is almost winter. I am ten.

I am looking at the door to my bedroom. The lights are on even though the whole house is asleep. There is no more wholeness in the house, just me and Grandmother. But we are the house. To my left is the wall, bumpy and painted blue. To my right is the edge of the bed, and if you step off without the right slipper socks, the aliens or sand monsters will get you. Behind me is my pillow, which is flat and covered in spots of blood. The air is dry, and my nose does not like that. So, blood spots. I am staring at the ceiling because I am inside. If I were outside, I would see the stars, and if I were near the house, I would see the roof. Below my feet is the other edge of my bed. There is a small pathway to the closet, and there you will find bags of Mother's clothes because plastic will keep them fresher, safe. They do not hang well anymore. Grandmother tore them all off their hangers on the one-year anniversary of Mother's disappearance. She left them in a heap. She placed them in storage bags the second year. Now I sit on them like bean bags. They keep my closet warm; they insulate.

I am a sad sack. Year three, soon. I don't know what Grandmother will do with Mother and Father's clothes. Grandmother knits only potholders because we have a lot of pots, and a lot to hold.

I am a sad sack, and Grandmother doesn't like to see it when she feels like a sad bag. Together we are just holding on.

Owl pulls a small object from her pocket, hands it to Sophie. "For the tofu and the telephone," she says.

Sophie takes the object, which turns out to be a plastic doll hand.

"I catch lots out there," says Owl. "Keep an old milk crate in my truck filled with this stuff."

Sophie turns the hand over and over, then tries to give it back to Owl. The woman holds up her own hand, shakes her head. Sophie places it besides the salt and pepper shakers, the tiny cracked fingers pointing out the peeling ceiling.

"So much from that tsunami in Japan finds its way here. I catch something new every time I fish. Normally I give it to the university. Nerds over there like studying these things." She pauses. "I don't get how they can just *study* these bits—just specks and pieces of people's lives—and not feel torn up inside. You know? But today, something told me to hang on to this one."

"Why?"

"I dunno. I have an eye like a hawk. A journalist is kind of like a hunter. And out there on the water, yesterday, a piece of chewed wood—probably from a boat or something. Or a clock. All this Japanese writing on it. Tomorrow, who knows? But today, this . . . small hand. Like the ocean was reaching out to me."

"What are you searching for?"

"I'm like that wife in Japan who has gone diving every day since the tsunami, searching for the bodies of her missing husband and daughter. She brings back to shore the broken dolls, chair legs, cooking pots, toaster ovens, tennis rackets, shoes of others who have gone missing. A total hodgepodge. You should see the piles.

Pillaged things . . . all mutts, just tails of wolves, mixed-up pieces. That woman, she dives every single day because she needs to do something. I'm like her. I like to put these pieces together, I love puzzles, the mystery, the selfishness, hunting for The Story."

Sophie imagines the diver discovering her husband and daughter on the dark ocean floor, seated at a kitchen table, chopsticks in hand, their bowls of noodles still full, her daughter's long black hair swirling around her head in the swift ocean current. "Will she ever find them?"

"What do you think?"

Sophie studies Owl, who has returned to investigating the bookshelf, pulling volumes out, running her fingers along the spines, and placing her nose in the creases. When Sophie goes to the kitchen for a glass of water, she checks her reflection in the window. She wishes that her elephant ears weren't quite so wrinkled, that her sleeve didn't have that charred spot from when she'd tried to make her mother's fried codfish recipe. She's glad that she's worn one of her mother's dress shirts underneath her elephant coat, though the green polyester blouse made her back sweat. When she serves more tea to Grandmother, she looks at the older woman's reflection in the window, marvels at Owl's sprightly posture compared to Grandmother's hunch.

"What about you?" Owl asks Grandmother.

"What about?"

"People in town say that you've kind of . . ." She points a finger at her own ear, makes a looping gesture. ". . . lost it."

Grandmother slurps her tea, eyes closed.

Sophie, nervous, tries to change the subject, asks, "When you're fishing, how do you know if what you're catching is just trash?"

Owl seems to think carefully about this. She goes on to describe her life as a journalist, her love of nature, how she likes to combine the two skills. She once stalked a wounded badger, followed its tracks for hours, her eyes on the ground, chin to chest, glasses slipping off the salt-grit sunblock on her nose. The badger made loops around trees, stopped to urinate on a mushroom. She describes how the mustelid's footprints became obscured by its low wide body, how when it got tired, its stomach dragged through the dirt, dusting its own overlapping pigeon-toed tracks. "But I still tracked him down. And I can make the distinction between what's trash and what's fodder. If it's not part of someone's life . . . well, let's just say that I can tell when something was thrown out, when they didn't want it anymore."

Grandmother scowls at this last comment, places her tea cup down with a loud *clack* on the table.

Owl checks her watch, scrutinizes the walls cluttered with photos of Sophie's parents and Grandmother. "Don't you ever want to get out of here? Out of this, um, *place*?"

"We are waiting," says Sophie.

"All you have here is . . . just waiting to get *old*. You've got brains, kid. You figured out this Braille stuff. You already know how to take care of . . ." She looks over at Grandmother. ". . . people and stuff."

Sophie shrugs awkwardly. She tries to serve Owl more tea.

The woman puts a hand over her cup. "If they wanted to come back, if they could, wouldn't they have?"

Sophie places the teapot down on the tray.

"How are you taking care of her? How did *they*? I couldn't do it. Come home every day after a long day at work to take care of someone else."

"It wasn't so bad. We were all together. We were like bees in our own little hive," says Sophie.

"Bees?"

"I knew how to take out the trash. I helped cook. I could clean Grandmother." Sophie remembers the story of the real hive that her mother grew up caring for on the roof of the public housing tenement that she and Grandmother and Grandfather once lived in. She tells Owl how bees sleep in cold weather, a full hive, thousands and thousands of bees clustered, cheek-to-cheek, in a tight ball. She describes the misunderstood anger of bees, their true gentle nature. And how when bees' wings get too old, those bees leave the hive and crawl around on the ground waiting to die, but that Sophie's mother would carefully pinch them between two fingers and place them on the lip of the hive box. She'd never been stung.

Sophie's parents drove a red Saab, thirty years old, purchased from an elderly barber who lived on their block. For weeks helicopters swept the beaches surrounding the small village, searching for a glimmer of its taillight or a sliver of bumper or hubcap, or a shredded tire floating in the low tide with a nail puncturing its rubber wall. But aside from the van full of tourists that plummeted from the cliffs one stormy night, there was no evidence of a crash.

Owl stops by Sophie's parents' bedroom on her way back from the bathroom, inspects the brocade bedspread, olive walls, a dresser displaying fox skulls, a raccoon skin, and a whole baby otter that they'd found washed up on the beach one January. The village taxidermist had tried to repair the tears in the forelegs and throat, wounds from a speedboat propeller or a battle with a predator as it plunge-dived for little sea creatures to eat, or when it crashed onto the rocky shore, its limp body riding the waves.

Sophie's mother once wrote down the recipe the taxidermist used for skins and furs inside the cover of her favorite cookbook:

Soaking, relaxing skin in salt
Fleshing, rendering off the remaining fat and muscle to get to
    the true skin
Currying, paring down the skin's thickness
Whizzing, extracting moisture in a salad spinner
Drumming, removing oil using hot, dry sawdust
Beating and beating and beating

Sophie describes to Owl running up to the dead animal; she remembers startling flocks of pipers and gulls so they squawked and looped overhead, her parents' excited shouts as she kicked up sand behind her.

"Why an elephant?" asks Owl. She starts nibbling her cold tofu cube, changes her mind and places it inside of a napkin that she balls in her fist.

Sophie describes her first morning as an elephant. The village doughnut shop. Wobbly gray paper ears stapled to a jogger's sweatband, long tube-sock trunk duct-taped to the end of her nose. Her tiny frame swimming in a voluminous gray wool coat. Face pressed against the finger-smudged glass case, fixated on a row of elephant doughnuts with white icing tusks and pink sprinkled earflaps. Inside the doughnut shop, the air boiled. Finger faces drawn on the fogged glass.

As far as Halloween costumes went, Sophie's was a sweaty disaster. But Grandmother, dressed as a ghost pirate with wide purple stripes and streaky maroon anchors drawn with lipstick on her wrinkly forearms, had announced proudly to the doughnutress how they had been up since four o'clock, costumed and seated at their kitchen table with mugs of hot tea to warm their hands. How they'd waited for sunrise, for the shop to open, how she was rewarding her granddaughter for her dedication to Halloween. Grandmother repeated the story to the other doughnut enthusiasts as they swarmed around the dynamic costumed duo, buzzing like mosquitoes: "How often do you get to dress up as what you most want to be?"

There were reports that Sophie's parents had been spotted in Boston. In San Francisco. In Virginia. In a tobacco shop in Georgia. Down at the Pak-n-Pay near the interstate. None of these were true, and Grandmother had long ago stopped reading the newspaper or answering phone calls from reporters seeking to confirm these false leads. "I'm tired of living in a fishbowl," she'd said to Sophie. "I don't know what else to tell them. What they're hunting for, I'm not sure. I'd rather go deaf and blind than listen to or read any more of this nonsense."

But Sophie didn't give up. She borrowed a police scanner from the same elderly barber who'd sold her parents the Saab. She set it up in the basement. At night, after the old woman went to sleep, Sophie tiptoed downstairs to listen to reports of cats stuck in trees, neighbors' heated disputes over fence lines, and men beating their wives and children and elderly parents. She felt like she was listening in on what her father called "taxicab secrets," which are very different from "barbershop secrets": One kind of secret you told knowing that the only thing the other person had on you was a rearview-mirror glimpse of the top of your forehead, while the other you told in a tiny room full of neighbors, understanding that your story would be mythologized and gossiped along, ear to ear, neighbor to neighbor, their *shhhhhh* as you entered a room sounding like an iron left on at full steam.

Listening to the scanner, Sophie would fall asleep and dream about the dark secrets of her village, oftentimes taking the dream form of a superheroine who could fly and turn invisible and breathe underwater and walk through her neighbors' walls to rescue the victims of bullies, young and old.

Sophie excuses herself, goes to the bathroom. As she washes her hands, she examines herself in the mirror. The tattered elephant ears. The soiled sweatband. The duct tape attaching the trunk has left a ridge of stickum, burnt umber lines across her nose that do not scrub off.

Sophie imagines Owl giving her a tour of the elegant institution where she works, its marble pillars and polished granite floors. The mechanical *korr-korr-arrrr* sounds of newspapers being printed echoing throughout the thirty-story building. For the tour, Sophie and Owl would wear matching structured mossy tweed dress-suits. Owl would introduce Sophie to her colleagues as her long-lost niece. Grandmother could be there, too. But just visiting, unpushy and whisper-quiet, giving everyone meaningful life lessons.

Owl and Sophie would have sophisticated chitchats about using coriander in recipes and dispense advice about where to find the best shoe cobblers in the city. And as they left the office, Owl's colleagues would wave purple streamers and spangle the air with ruby glitter like professional funeral wailers, mourn and gossip after Sophie and Owl's grand departure. Once outside on the bright sidewalk, Sophie would be greeted by her parents, who had been waiting forever for her, wondering why it took her so long, and saying didn't she look dapper and so grown up, and what a ladylike haircut, and asking how *is* everyone back in the village, and complimenting her on taking such good care of herself.

Sophie shivers as she thinks of big city life for an elephant, of her trumpeting debut independence.

The last person to see Sophie's parents was the graveyard-shift janitor, Ed Root, a private man with a bright funny face, known by the staff as the human radio because he sang along to tunes that he made up, in a voice like a saw.

Did they say anything? Did they seem distressed? The newspapers had reported the sheriff's questions to the janitor. *Had either of them been drinking? Was there any indication that they were trying to flee something or someone?*

Sophie has always imagined her parents asking the janitor for help in jump-starting their Saab before heading home. While the man untangled cables, fiddled with tubes and knobs under the hoods of their two cars, her parents probably told him jokes, about paying him a thousand dollars to brush their teeth for them, wash their hair, change them into flannel pajamas, carry them upstairs to bed, tuck them in with two fingers of whiskey for each. For an extra thousand, they'd love to have him use his scratching, gurgling voice to read their daughter to sleep from her favorite book about magical talking bears, to sing her one of his made-up songs, something that sounded like *hoo-ooo owl, ow-owly, owly, ah ah ah.* Her parents were still wearing their nursing uniforms: Mother's womb-red, soft; Father's teal, stained, worn thin at the ankle hem. Their matching brown leather clogs resounded, clomping through the underground garage like a pair of tired horses, forty-eight-hour-shift tired.

Owl checks her watch. "It's getting late. What could possibly take him this long? Do I need to go into town and drag the mechanic here myself?"

"He is the only one. *And* the managing janitor for the hospital *and* middle school *and* the mayor—" says Grandmother.

"—the *deputy* mayor," Sophie chimes in.

"I can't wait all day. I'm a problem solver. This is ridiculous." Owl glances around the room, and then at Sophie. "Why don't you give me your phone number? I'd love to call you when I'm back in the city. Would you want to visit?"

Sophie looks eagerly at Grandmother, who remains perfectly still, her expression unreadable. The waning afternoon light brings out the faded everything in the room; the navy walls, so regal when her parents had first painted them, now just seem too harsh for such a small space.

"I don't want to take you away. You could come just for a visit, maybe even visit the office. Everyone would love to meet you," says Owl, looking between Sophie and Grandmother. When Sophie does not chirp up, Owl becomes impatient, frowns. "Look, just write your phone number down and we'll figure something out."

Sophie looks around the living room for a scrap to write on. She checks the junk drawer, behind the coin bowl where they normally keep a small stack of mail they haven't read. Owl taps her foot, and Sophie becomes afraid that Owl will leave if she doesn't solve this paper dilemma fast enough. Again she pictures her glittery life in the big city, the hurried steps she'll take to keep up with Owl's long strides, her tweedy arrival at the newspaper office.

Slowly, Sophie tears one elephant ear from her head, the paper worn, yielding, with edges that feel like soft cotton wonder. She hopes her parents will forgive her, hopes they will be able to recognize her with just one ear, just half the elephant that remembers them. Writing her phone number—her very first phone number, her first memorized thing—in thick block numbers with an inky black pen on the creased gray construction paper, she hands it to Owl. But Grandmother reaches out, stabbing the air with her wrinkled, knobby fingers, trying to snatch it.

"She's giving it to me!" says Owl.

"You leave her be. You leave!" says Grandmother.

"I can make up my own mind, Grandma," says Sophie.

Grandmother and Owl tussle for a moment, the older woman straining to grab the ear out of the other's hand, but the fisherwoman holds her off easily with one arm. Sophie almost laughs at the scene, though the walls of the room seem to tighten as she watches the two women spar over her elephant ear.

Owl: her arm outstretched, palm to Grandmother's forehead.

Grandmother: swinging at the empty air between her and Owl. And her hair, which normally holds the curls from the same set of aluminum curlers she has slept in since the 1920s, has become unraveled so that pieces stick up like silver antennae.

Owl, who is not wearing shoes, who looks like she's never walked anywhere without shoes, braces herself by trying to dig her toes into the linoleum.

As their standoff continues, Sophie is struck by how, now that it is no longer stapled to her head, her ear looks just like a tattered piece of paper. The other one, still attached, dangles by the metal prong of a staple. The block numbers she'd written so carefully around the curve of the ear have bled through the paper in places where it is irreparably creased.

Sophie's chair scrapes the floor as she stands. Worried that her grandmother will hurt herself, Sophie tries to wedge between the two women, but Owl easily pushes the girl away so that Sophie stumbles backward.

"You're crazy! You are both crazy!" Owl is out of breath, eyebrows knitted. "Can't you see what you're doing to this girl?" she says to Grandmother. "Indulging her! Letting her stink in this saltbox shithole! In that ridiculous costume! You are destroying her life! I don't care if you've lost your marbles or not. I don't care if you can hear me or not. The people in the village are right. You two are just going to rot away here. Just waiting waiting waiting. For *what*?"

Grandmother blinks.

Owl huffs a sigh and begins to gather her things. Sophie realizes that the woman does not care enough about either of them to keep fighting.

Sophie helps Grandmother sit back down; the old woman is panting, red-faced, but with a strangely calm expression. Sophie observes the mouths of the women: one agape and resolute, and the other scowling.

Sophie's last driving trip with her mother was to shop in the city for her annual first-day-back-to-school dress. The freshly washed Saab stalled in a busy downtown intersection, like a bright red apple blocking traffic, cars honking, arms waving out of open windows, and her mother's scratchy old-school music blaring on the radio—a nasal, wheezy, chanting flight-song:

> *Apple-cherry-apple pie!*
> *Better than the sweetest tea!*
> *Come join me, join me! Have a try!*
> *The nicest time to bee-eeeee!*

"Don't worry about sounding lo-fi," her mother said to Sophie over the din. "Just don't go through life jaded. I'm not talking the smoking cigarettes—but don't you smoke, Sophie!—and sitting in a café kind. But the wearing leather that you hate because you're not comfortable in your own skin kind." She smiled at Sophie, gave her earlobe a tug. "Know what to reach for and figure out where to find it." She reached across the space in front of Sophie, knocking into the spruce green thermos of coffee with her elbow, stretched her arm out of her daughter's window, and with a belligerent scowl, warm cheeks, she flipped off cars and people in the intersection, honkers or not, to their right, left, and straight ahead (*Fuck fuck fuck!*).

Owl gathers her tackle box and her rod from the front hall. The curtains in the living room, midnight purple, rustle in the wind brought in by the open door. As the fisherwoman puts on her rubber boots, leaning to tuck her jeans into the tops, the gray paper ear with Sophie's phone number falls out of her pocket. Neither Owl nor Grandmother sees it. Sophie does not pick it up; instead, she follows the woman out the front door, stands on the top step, and watches as Owl strides down the road, head bent against the wind, rod and tackle box gripped in hand, digging in her heels as she marches toward town.

Sophie Chu's Journal: Red Saab. I am in the backseat, playing rubber bands, but the bouncing makes me carsick. I face the horizon because this will cure me. Colors of dawn:

> *Blue*
> *Blue*
> *Orange*
> *Red*
> *Purple*
> *Blue*

Inside the car it smells like coffee. The thermos steam swirls and curls, and it is all that I need in the world. Mother and Father are in the front. Mother is driving. It is autumn, so the reds are redder, or-anges brighter, yellows are golden. Everything is more. I am six in this memory, tall enough to rest my chin on the side door lip.

In front of me is the back of Father's head; salt and pepper, coarse, slicked back hard and full of crunch. To my left is an empty seat, but I have my pillow for when I want to stretch out to sleep.

Behind me is the road, dusty and forgotten. A pinpoint of black, reaching back back back. And right around the rear of the car, it glows red.

The upholstery peels away from the car's metal skull. Inside it is called the ceiling, Father explains. Outside, it is the roof. Inside is the floor. Outside is the ground. There's a difference, he says. Distinctions matter, he says.

Below my feet are crumbs, and my unlaced shoes, side by side. I am wearing socks. There are balls of Kleenex. The car is hush hush hush because it is morning. The carpet keeps it hushed. Gravel vibrates below the tires.

I am waiting. That is what it is to sit in a moving car. I am not di-recting. I am not driving. And that is okay. All you have to do is sit back and enjoy the ride. Relax, Mother says. We'll be there in no time.

In the break room at the village hospital, a man and woman stood at adjoining lockers. There were pumpkin decorations on the break room walls, layered over faded Christmas tree cutouts and Easter bunnies made by children in the pediatric cancer ward. Taped inside his locker, the man kept a poster of a nimble cat dangling from a branch, the words *Hang in There* printed across its face in bright yellow letters.

The woman rolled her eyes amiably every time she saw this. In her own locker, a photo of a girl about six years old, wickedly long black hair tangled all over the place. She reminded herself to be kinder to their daughter; she would not chide her to brush her teeth, would let her have one night of cavity-sweet dreams. She quickly scanned the empty room, wanted to kiss the man's salty cheek, taste his sweat from working a nearly completed triple-shift alongside her. The man wanted to rest his head for a moment on the woman's shoulder, his nose facing her neck, take in the worn cottony scent of her scrubs, hints of the sweet figs and savory olives she'd scarfed during their only break. The woman's stomach growled, and she thought about the midnight breakfast she'd cook for them before crashing into bed: eggs, whisk-beaten, scrambled fluffy so that they're lighter than air. And paper-thin potato slices fried in the pan, the starchy crisps served with dollops of sour cream and sprinkled with chopped scallions.

The woman wanted to whisper something into the man's ear to make his earlobes tremble; she thought of how arachnids rub silky filaments between two legs, musical vibrations to attract other spiders, a sound that she's always imagined was like a mourning dove's deep rolling purr: *coo, coo-curroo coo-curroo, coo-coo-coooo*, a spider love song.

They left the break room, headed back out into the bright hallway, ready to complete their final rounds. Both wanted to squeeze the other's fingers, a secret handshake of knowing. Later there would be time. The blue light buzzed, an orderly rushed past with a gurney whose wheels pinched their eardrums with *skwee-skwee-skwee*, and their shifts groaned on.

THIS IS ME

Mrs. Lee is in the middle of her third cup of tea when Grace strides into her kitchen, a handkerchief held to her mouth.

"You're here. Must be Sunday," says Mrs. Lee, seated at the table in front of a small television. She peers up at her seventy-year-old daughter, studies the blunt shape of Grace's expensive haircut, the sheerness of her white linen sleeveless top, the suppleness of her orange leather purse. "What is a dying person like?"

"The tar! How can they do street work in this heat?" Grace surveys the small room: the pale-blue walls, the crocheted curtain over the kitchen sink, the high-tech soap dispenser she had given her mother on her ninetieth birthday, the glass mixing bowl in which a single white fish floats like a lazy ghost, the moving boxes of dishes that Grace had begun packing the week earlier, and the food-encrusted dinner plates from the night before.

"What is a dying person like?" repeats Mrs. Lee.

Grace exhales loudly, shakes her head. "Nobody's dying. Where's Dad?"

"Your dad starts at four o'clock this morning. So I start at four o'clock." Mrs. Lee accepts a hug from her daughter, studies her. Always there are those sharp-eyed spiders, she thinks. Eyes on everybody, legs on everything; these are the bugs that she steers clear of. For her, the slow movement and shimmering scales and round elegant body of a Moonlight Gourami is ideal. She will let herself be happily mesmerized for hours by her pet fish, its looping travels.

"Aren't you hot in that? It's a hundred degrees out!" Grace tries to roll up her mother's sleeves, but Mrs. Lee swats at her hands. "Have you been outside today? Where is Mimi? Why is all this out here? You have to tell her to do these things, Mom. That's what you pay her for."

Mrs. Lee lifts her chin. The small white hairs on her knuckles bristle at her daughter's efficiency.

Grace pulls a banana from her purse and drops it on the table, says, "And we are not moving this fridge. This is a piece of garbage." With a beet-stained sponge, she wipes a small puddle that has formed at the base of the leaky appliance, then with damp hands begins to strip the fridge of the photos that papered its metal front, carelessly tossing them and the farm-animal magnets into a shoe box.

Mrs. Lee imagines the colors in the wet photographs bleeding together, the corners curling. She imagines waking up the next morning, the light crawling across the linoleum floor. She imagines her eyes finding the box—broken, soggy cardboard. She imagines falling on her aching knees, digging frantically through the photos to get to the bottom, where it is wettest. She imagines finding the most damaged photo and thinking how easy it would be, with the paper this wet, to tear it in half. An unwelcome yet irrepressible thought—like how everyone, when they walk on a tall bridge, thinks for just a split second what it would be like to jump.

"Well? Did you tell Mimi?" asks Grace, who has now begun pulling baking supplies out of the cupboards and setting them in the box on top of the photos.

"I fired her," says Mrs. Lee with a smile.

"Yes, I know. You can't keep firing her." Grace lets a cupboard door shut itself with a loud clack.

Mrs. Lee checks the kitchen clock. She waves her daughter over to the table. "My show starts now! Are you glued to the floor? Come on!" She turns on the television; the sounds of clapping and a cheerful announcer fill the kitchen. Grace's purse slides off the chair to the floor. Mrs. Lee glances suspiciously at the papers and brochures spilling out. On the TV, a woman bursts into tears as an announcer hands her a large purple vacuum; her entire family swarms the stage and engulfs her in a hug, arms squeezing and hands patting each other.

"Such a family," says Mrs. Lee. She is surprised when Grace starts to laugh. Mrs. Lee thinks of telling her daughter about Mimi's lurid boast the night before, of knowing one hundred ways to please a man. She thinks of telling how Mimi's good pay makes the forty-year-old Chinese woman lazy, clumsy, her head and canta-loupe breasts so big they seem to crash into everything, making the house seem smaller and smaller over the months since Mr. Lee's accident.

"Hurry, my show's starting." Mrs. Lee pats the chair next to her.

"First, tell me who's dying," responds Grace. The handsome announcer, a white man flashing white teeth, unveils a new vac-uum, twice the size of the previous one. Silver and sleek black, the vacuum reminds Mrs. Lee of the car that dropped her caretaker off on her first day of work. She wonders who the driver had been, and why Mimi never speaks of the glamorous home that her pay-checks must surely be paying for.

As the vacuum on the television zooms across the stage, de-vouring an enormous pile of dried pinto beans, Mrs. Lee blurts out, "Your dad says he's dying."

"Why?" Grace, alarmed, turns to her mother.

"I'll tell you later." Mrs. Lee does not take her eyes off the tele-vision.

Grace squeezes her mother's arm as she brushes past. "I'm going to check on Dad."

Last year, after Mr. Lee slipped in the shower, Grace had found her mother spoon-feeding him rice porridge. At the time, he was seated on the bathroom floor, a towel rolled and placed behind his back, another towel draped over his shoulders for warmth, his lucky blue pajamas yanked clumsily over his bony hips, which were bruised deep-green and purple. For three days, Mrs. Lee had eaten and slept in the bathroom alongside her husband. She was unable to move him, and she was too proud to call her daughter or Mimi for help. Grace had decided then that Mimi would come seven days a week instead of two, at hours that never seemed to be the same from one day to the next. Grace decided how much more to pay her. Grace decided the color of Mr. Lee's new pajamas. Grace had decided a lot of things, and Mrs. Lee had wondered what she and her husband were becoming: not parents, not children—but a bump on the head, interior deadbolts that required Grace's or Mimi's key to open, a liability.

Mrs. Lee hears her daughter's returning footsteps and turns up the volume of the television.

Grace drops into a seat beside her mother. "He looks good in red."

"He doesn't like red. But Mimi. Always, red red red."

"Where's Mimi? Why isn't she here yet? I just talked to her on the phone."

"I told you. I fired her! I fire her, and she always shows up. And my fish food, missing. Your dad's diapers, missing."

"Nobody is stealing," sighs Grace.

"I tell you. I will catch Mimi in action, and then I will fire her and call the police at the same time."

Grace squints at the TV. "What is this?"

"This is the longest commercial. I want to go crazy."

"I think this is an infomercial."

Mrs. Lee and Grace watch as the announcer shouts a play-by-play like a sportscaster as two audience members, each armed with a different vacuum, race to vacuum up mounds of glittering paperclips poured onto the stage.

"What's the difference between those vacuums?" asks Grace.

"About ten dollars. Anyway, I'm thinking. Why don't we move in with you? Your place is so big I can hear echoes." Mrs. Lee actually cannot remember Grace's grand lakeside apartment but imagines slick marble counters, plush carpets, and elegant vertical blinds like the ones she's seen in movies.

"You are going to a new place. Remember?" Grace pulls out a stack of papers with photos of smiling elderly white people. "Please, Mom. Look at the brochure again. This is where you are going."

Mrs. Lee ignores her daughter, runs her hand admiringly across the purse's leather.

"It's a knock-off," says Grace flatly.

Mrs. Lee's sharp brown eyes search Grace's face. She has tried to understand the whole hush-hush world of business and medicine that her daughter is always prescribing. Grace's cell phone rings; she picks it up to see who is calling, then drops it back on the table without answering.

"Are you mad at everyone?" asks Mrs. Lee.

"No, just you," says Grace with a smile. She picks up her phone again, taps the screen and begins to listen to a voicemail. She nods her head to the chattering in her ear and begins to fill a moving box with her mother's rice bowls, wrapping them in faded dish towels. The sound reminds Mrs. Lee of the chattering birds in the early mornings when her husband's whimpering wakes her, when she tiptoes across the hallway to spy in the dark, finding Mimi seated at the edge of Mr. Lee's bed, wiping his mouth with a tissue—the grateful nodding, the low murmurs, Mimi patting Mr. Lee's trembling hand.

"You talk to Mimi, everyone, but not me." Mrs. Lee draws an

X across her lips with a finger. "You always have secrets. What's wrong with telling me?"

Grace slides the brochure for Two Star Senior Park over to her mother, stuffs a new box with crumpled newspaper, padding the bottom, then opens the cabinet containing large platters and pie dishes.

"Why two stars? Why not four?" Mrs. Lee squints at the elegant black man and woman holding hands and grinning as they walk toward a young Asian woman in a white uniform, standing in the middle of a small gray room, holding a large tray of drinks and orange pill bottles. Though their hair is white, the couple's unlined faces do not look much older than her daughter's. Mrs. Lee shakes her head. "Your dad doesn't know I'm here."

"You'll have friends to gossip with." Grace kneels beside the box, her face red from the heat and the uncomfortable position.

"Only gossip about who's dying next." Mrs. Lee wriggles her fingers. "I have pain all over."

"I fought for you and Dad to have the best room. The biggest. Lots of sunlight. Everything."

"You always love shopping. Buy this and that. Not make-do."

"I make do. This IS making do!"

Mrs. Lee examines the spots on her hand, bends and straightens fingers as knobby as a pear tree's branches. She thinks of her family's ancient pear tree but cannot remember why, at the age of eight, she had protested the cutting of the tree, even though it was mostly stripped of its bark and leaves by beetles and rot. She had dangled from the topmost branch like a limp noodle while Eldest Brother, nearly twenty years her senior, ax in hand, stared at her from their family's courtyard below.

For years she had asked herself the same questions: why didn't her parents scream when the Communist soldiers stormed through their home, tore up paintings, burned scrolls detailing her family's lineage through the last two dynasties? How could her parents watch as their eldest son was dragged away, hands bound, a wooden pole and red flag of shame the size of a napkin waving above his head? Why did Eldest Brother, a poet and teacher, kill himself when he returned home, weeks after her parents had paid a hefty bribe? Why did the "official" documents, signed by her parents, list the cause of her brother's death as "richness and boredom"?

Mrs. Lee tries to recall Eldest Brother's eyes from the weeks before his imprisonment, to remember whether they had held any sympathy for her predicament in the tree, but all she can recall is the smell of sweet white blossoms crushed beneath her fingers, the roughness of the bark digging into her palms as she hung, wilted, legs flapping in the empty space.

"Have you been taking the medicine Dr. Wong prescribed?" Grace begins packing up the canned vegetables, the jars of pickled meats, and jugs of canola oil.

"I tell you," responds Mrs. Lee, "your grandmother, grandfather, uncles. We once lived in what you call a palace. I don't know if you believe. We had a pantry just for fruit! We had a white tile floor, the wall, everything. So elegant. It was so beautiful. Even the watermelon looked new."

"You don't need white tile. Fruit pantries. A palace. You can just do this . . . for Dad, for me."

"You don't know anything."

"Rrrrraaaa! I'm doing all of this for you!"

"Stop this *rraa*. Don't get yourself all crazy."

Grace looks at her watch. "Where is Mimi? I can't believe this heat. Aren't you hot in that?" She wipes her forehead with her handkerchief.

"Mimi is no good. I tell her, 'Don't do this, don't do that.' Repeat and repeat again." Mrs. Lee taps her temple with an index finger. "Kind of dumb."

Grace takes a break to eat her banana. She makes a face when she bites into the fruit, which has a large brown splotch hidden beneath the peel. "Two Star has dozens of helpers, smart ones."

Mrs. Lee studies the column of mixing bowls nested, one inside the other, on the counter beside the enormous fish bowl. She wonders if Grace can see that the fish, though white and spectral, is still living and breathing and circling inside the most comfortable bowl.

"I'm checking on Dad." Grace tosses the half-eaten banana on the table.

Mrs. Lee's nose follows Grace's sweaty trail: a blend of flowery deodorant and burnt wood and irritation. She waits until she can no longer hear her daughter's footsteps, then grabs the remote and turns the volume way up. The television announcer is vacuuming a small hill of sand to demonstrate the machine's suction power. The whirring motor sounds like it is wheezing. Mrs. Lee fans herself with one of the brochures. She nibbles the bruised banana, lets the sour pulp squeeze between her gums and loose dentures—a glue, ripening, something sweet for her to find later. She cannot remember if Grace has always acted like this, or whether her concern had magnified because of Mr. Lee's accident—when the police found him alone, haunting the hilly streets near their house, with bare feet cut and bloody, a strange bump on his head. Earlier, Mrs. Lee had used animated arms to describe to the policeman her husband's mysterious disappearance. He'd been missing for many hours, maybe the whole day, Mrs. Lee explained as she pointed to an imaginary sun as it passed over the sky, rising then setting. If it had been herself who was lost, she had boasted, she would follow the sun, and then she would be home.

Mrs. Lee glances at the clock. Almost time. She dreads the sounds of Mimi's keys jangling in the front door, the dropping of her heavy shoes on the floor with a clunk-clunk. Grace will go to greet her, and Mrs. Lee will try to decipher their murmurs, tilting her head, hoping to capture the secret in her ears. The brave buzz of vacuums and cheering on the television will join Mimi's clumsy noises. Mimi will check on Mr. Lee first, find him waiting for her, his bedroom heavy with wet diaper and nightmares and red. Mimi will clean him, then begin to pack his room, throwing heavy books into boxes, wrapping dusty clocks in Mr. Lee's whitest shirts.

Grace returns, takes a gulp of tea, settles herself in a chair, and clears her throat. "Look . . . someone's coming tomorrow. My friend. A lawyer. She specializes in . . . handling things like this. Remember, I have power of attorney."

"Why is that you always get the power? You be our boss? You let your dad make up his mind."

"He doesn't have any mind left!"

Mrs. Lee does not recognize the wobble in Grace's voice, a wet sound, unstable, like she's swallowing raw egg yolk. "He's able to do, you know, some things. Sometimes good, sometimes not too good."

"What are you talking about?"

"You're in cahoots! You and your lawyer and dumb Mimi . . . Are you better than me? I ask you."

"Do you even remember what you ate for breakfast today?"

"Last night at dinner, he tells me he's dying. I heat up my noodles, but he does not want to eat. But then he watches me eat and eat, and he must smell it, because he goes to his bowl and even though his noodle was cold, your dad, he . . ." Mrs. Lee shovels imaginary food into her mouth with finger chopsticks, and makes bulldozer sounds. "And I think . . . if he was dying, he wouldn't eat like that."

Grace leans in. "When you move, you'll get to fire Mimi."

Mrs. Lee tries to think seriously about this, but at first finds herself thinking in numbers: number of curse words she has shouted at her dreaming husband, number of resentments expressed in crude jokes, number of commands she's given Mimi, number of hours searching for lost eyeglasses, number of nightmares, number of years since her father and mother and brothers died, number of times she has thought of them with fondness and anger and tears.

"Mom. Mom? Are you listening? I said that you'll get to fire Mimi when you move to Two Star."

Mrs. Lee imagines what it would be like sharing a studio apartment like the one in the brochure, one room, no more space for shadows and ghosts: she could no longer disobey her daughter's rules, fire Mimi. She tries to imagine what it would be like to watch TV without Mimi to distract her, but she cannot picture a life watching TV somewhere that isn't home, in a place where a hundred Mimis will order her around. She can't imagine taking her last breath surrounded by strangers she does not care to know. She wonders what it would take to convince Grace, and decides to let her generosity shine through: "Where else can a dumb person go? I feel bad."

"I am going to finish packing the books." Grace touches her mother's arm and starts to leave the room.

"Did I tell you? Last week I go to market to buy more bananas. There was a gunshot! People yelling, crying, Mimi hiding. I keep shopping, picking fruit. I mean, what can you do? And I ask her, 'Are you afraid to die?'"

"Jesus! Why didn't you hide?" Grace covers her eyes with her hands and laughs despite herself.

"No, I tell you! Don't hide. That's terrible. And, anyway, why are you so tense? Why give yourself so much pressure?"

"Please, just . . . This facility is amazing. There are ice cream socials. And you don't have to shop for yourself or even leave your bed. Life will just come to you."

Mrs. Lee watches her daughter's movements—jumpy, hungry, a kicking and pecking pigeon. She pushes the papers away. "What life is that? Just lying there, waiting to die?"

"Mom."

Mrs. Lee turns to watch a woman on the television, one wearing a headset and racing frantically onto the stage to unplug the vacuum just as the announcer steers it into a puddle of water. "I feel good. The bad part is your dad's brain. I feel, how could I say, I feel . . . I help him to go."

Grace grabs the remote and turns off the TV. "By yourself here, you'd go completely nuts."

Desperate to see what has become of the announcer, Mrs. Lee reaches for Grace's hand, which still clutches the remote. "Your dad and me. Once we visited a new place, a place for old turtles like us."

"And? I bet you it was great!" Grace throws her arms up in the air.

"I tell you. I take one look around and think two words." Mrs. Lee raises a knobby, arthritic finger in the air like a snake that's just swallowed an egg. "Not enough." She pictures the single room, the bright fluorescent glare, the sensible safety bars, the plush berber carpet. "So, why do I want to do that? More brave to live here, my own way. These walls, I know. This table—" She knocks the table with her knuckles. "—I know."

"Brave? Because you live where people shoot other people while you're buying bananas?"

She wonders why her daughter would prefer for her to live in a world of brightness and bars and berber, when she could lurk in the corners of her own home like a ghost, haunting herself and Mr. Lee whenever she wanted. At home she could sink into a different deep wingback chair in each room, to hide from Mimi, at least for a minute. At home she could sit in the living room and stare across the length of the hallway and see the doorway to every room she and Mr. Lee had decorated together, each panel of blue wallpaper they'd unrolled and hung sixty years ago. And from her favorite chair near the front door, she could watch the world through the wavy glass window that had been cracked when Grace had taught herself, as a girl, to roller skate inside the house. She knows each room she and her husband made love in to celebrate their different anniversaries in their first years in the house together. She knows each door they slammed during fights. Each broken thing, each speck of dust, each spider web, each creak in the wide-planked oak floor, is hers.

Where would her spirit go if she died in Two Star? Every day, to an ice cream social? Then to bed with no memories to surround her? Mrs. Lee turns to talk to the dark television screen. "I wonder if they see me watching them, think I have all the answers?"

Grace watches her mother with the same expression she'd had when she'd bitten into the bad banana.

Mrs. Lee loudly asks the television, "Can you see me? I'm watching you!"

Grace shakes her head sharply. "Mom! You're talking to the TV. And it's not even on!"

Mrs. Lee turns the television back on, points to the screen while facing Grace. "Look, see all these winners? Everyone cheering! The big lights! Vacuums! So many treasures! There's no better place except—" Mrs. Lee looks proudly around her small blue kitchen. "—maybe here. This is *me*."

"Packing is almost finished. Mom. Do you understand?"

Mrs. Lee ponders her daughter's question as her tongue digs for banana in the plastic grooves of her dentures; she tastes sourness, a secret fear. For a moment, Mrs. Lee imagines herself as a turtle—not snapping or giant—but with a pale underbelly, a shell not hard enough to protect her when children kick her down the road.

She observes the way the light from the kitchen window reflects off the wetness of her daughter's eyes; the brown irises, solid wood walls encased by two smaller bright white windows. "Tell me, you know, what you're thinking."

The windows dim for a moment, and Mrs. Lee's breath catches. Where has she seen this before? She scours her memories, running along the grooves of her brain, searching in all the darkest corners until she finally meets Eldest Brother. Is this a dream? Is this a vision? Who is to say? But Mrs. Lee can finally remember Eldest

Brother's eyes: two polished chestnuts, shining, unblinking as they furiously scan the pear tree trunk, the pebbled ground, the white sky, in search of the wings or cloud that had lifted his baby sister to the top of the dying tree. She hears the sound of Eldest Brother's hand sliding along the rough silver-colored bark, probing, measuring the few remaining limbs. She watches as he tests the sharpness of the ax's blade with his thumb. Eldest Brother staggers under the weight of each cut branch, feeding them into the small fire he's made. Mrs. Lee wonders: how much will Eldest Brother cut before she must drop?

ANATOMY OF A CLOUD

The low sunrise, seeping through mist, glows from the mountain cave opening. Fei slowly waves her paw, cuts the air above Ying-Long's face, a shadow to wake him. She circles the hard ground where he lies. YingLong's breath is staggered, no longer able to form clouds to soak the mountain region, nor fog, thick around the mountain's neck. Imagine: air in, snow out. Fei checks for the tiny hearts that should beat in his paws, throat, and chest. Ying-Long, the last dragon god of rain, does not stir.

Fei bows her head, her long leathery wings folded and resting neatly on her ridged back so that they do not drag on the dusty ground. She listens to YingLong's breaths, the rattling *ch ch ch ch* sound of thirsty clouds. Biological burble. She walks like YingLong once flew, swerving left and right. She studies his brilliant blue scars, wounds from dry lightning strikes—like shafts of sun and *yún*, like virga, like crystal storm sublime—where the azure tear-drop scales would not regenerate on the back of his slender neck.

When YingLong's father died, Fei had been diligently working on her clay sculpture by the nearly dry riverbed. When she sculpts, she cannot hear the carrion crows cawing or the cockroaches' gregarious chirping. Her thoughts are so loud, the only other sound is of her claw scraping designs and shaping the deep red clay. When she returned on that day to their mountaintop dwelling and found YingLong, she had thought that his paleness and hunch were for her. She observed the artifacts scattered around YingLong's feet: a chicken-claw back scratcher; a sand dollar that YingLong had carried home, tucked inside his cheek, from his final journey to his father's lonely mountain; an enchanted urn filled with precious water collected from clouds long ago. She understood then that they were now alone. When YingLong dies, Fei will be the last dragon. A coin without country, a book without pages. A name without meaning. A land without home.

Fei uses the chicken claw to comb YingLong's coarse beard, and recites stories of the afterworld, a place not deadened by drought, with oil slicks for oceans, black and mystery deep. Fei shakes the sand dollar to hear the sand inside. She puts it to her ear and listens to the grains slide over themselves, washing over rocks and sea ledges the way water once washed over the long-dead sharks and penguins, seaweed and jellyfish. The sand dollar lets her see underneath the beach. And there she finds millennia before the Anthropocene dried up the planet. She finds buried treasure, gold booty and purple gemstones, lost eyepatches of pirates. She finds the footsteps of every creature that has ever walked the beach, every bird, every warrior. She finds every seal and whale and dragon skeleton. She finds broken kite strings, lost tennis balls. She finds the ocean that was once glacier and once in Africa and on the cap of the earth.

As Fei braids YingLong's silver mane, she thinks back to her first attempt at flying as a juvenile. No mother to teach her. And father, long dead. So imagine the flailing wings, around and around. Never lifting off the ground. Dirt flinging everywhere, spoons- and shovelsful. And because her wings were not strong enough to lift her, she'd decided then to dig. With her lantern eyes at night. Yellow, brilliant blasts. She dug until her claws cracked and bled, to the same depths as the deepest ocean trench. And there, curled into a circle, she slept, dreamt of steam vents, fire and lava, krill and glowing fishes, of cures for every disease but the drought that ravaged the planet. She dreamt of lost civilizations, crashed airplanes and sunken boats. There, at the bottom of her sleeping ocean, in the darkest crevice of the earth, there were no shadows.

Fei and YingLong had shared a balloon-soft belief that the clay beast she sculpted would bring the desperately needed rain to the land. That the beast would have YingLong's gift of flight, that its arms, spread wide, would hold up the sky like caryatids, raising the planet's waters. But the night of YingLong's father's death: doubt, hard as wood. Loud as a rifle blast. Living lunacy. Fei remembers the sounds of sorrow that bled out of YingLong's horn mouth, mournful music that drowned and boomed, trumpet call for other dragons to join. But theirs were the only sounds. Their tears thickened with dirt. By morning, they'd used their claws to dig out the dried-tea-leaf dreams from the corners of their eyes.

Fei remembers the summer day she started the sculpture. After a long frigid winter, she'd been craving jasmine blossoms, which is the scent of dragons in love. The only scent that makes her scales glitter, lifts them from her body like fish gills—open and close and open and close. For many months, the mountain villagers had burned huge bonfire shrines in desperation, filling the sky with ash and prayers, calling out to the dragons for the rain they had not seen in ten years. As YingLong tried to gather the strength to fly again, Fei had descended the mountain, out of the choking smoke, and headed toward the river valley.

Fei started by building the beast's armature with elephant bones melded with fire and affixed with wax and tallow. She stuffed the frame with ostrich nests and juniper treetops. She built the wings many times larger than YingLong's, and extended them beyond the reaches of the valley. She molded armfuls of clay around this frame, slowly adding girth when she could find enough water. Fei's sculpture, a creature she and YingLong had dreamed about, was barn big with matted fur and a hinged metal jaw, its tongue a crimson belt beneath jagged teeth that grind and crunch. Exposed brain grooves like walnuts. A bony spine.

The villagers were in on it. They'd watched for weeks from across the valley, at first hidden in the shadows of trees at the edge of the forest, as Fei built her sculpture. The stories they were raised on as children, passed from generation to generation, taught them that this was the time to dip into their meager stores and give what they could if they were to survive. So they pooled together their resources and collected hundreds of elephant hides, massaging them every day with the last of their precious almond oil, so that the skin could stretch and double in size. Sons cut and braided a mile of ribbon made out of their fathers' long hair. Daughters and mothers stitched together the elephant hides—enough skin to wrap around the breadth of the sculpture. Without ceremony, they left their offerings at its base one night, after Fei had returned to her cave. In the morning, Fei found the villagers' gifts and let out a whooping cry of thanks, which from dragons sounds like a crack of thunder.

She attached the hide with thorns. Confident that her creation would be strong in its new skin, she gave her sculpture heavy rounded legs, like four oval pillars. The wind blew across the valley, bringing a cheerful murmur that sounded of the villagers' grief mixed with hope. She flapped her own misshapen wings, sending a blustery burst of air full of yellow pollen. She stood back and admired her work: She buried her snout in the sculpture's mane and almond skin, tested the wooden wings, the tightened bolts. Solid, swiveling. Certified beast.

Unlike YingLong, who is deaf, Fei hears everything, even sounds not yet made. She knew that the clay beast's talk would be garbled. Unlike the harsh words screamed at the sky, resounding with the villagers' growing desperation, beast speech was all vowels, no hard angles, heard low beneath the warble symphony, morning chorus. Fei carved a slit, crooked and ragged, where sounds would come from. Sounds like sand sliding over round river stones. Sounds like the final breath of an oak, decayed wood a shadow tree on the ground. Sounds like a moth rustling its wings, or ants scurrying and scurrying. Like the laying of an egg, or limbs growing inside a womb. Like fungus breaking earth, or snakes dragging trails in the dirt. Sounds of sun rising, the moon setting.

So different were these from the sounds of dragons in *love*. Imagine: long ago, the villagers chanting loudly, their necks cranked toward the sky. YingLong carrying Fei into the air, tangling them together, coiling tail to nose tip, rippling the clouds. The adults cheering with glee and understanding, and the children shouting at what they believed to be two deities battling one another: *Go, Big Vicious! Go, Big Vicious! Yes yes yes!* Pungent summer days, like fish oil over a fire, like steam rising off of damp dirt, like turtles swimming, their bubbles rising.

Fei ventures out of her mountain cave when she can no longer bear listening to YingLong's shallow bird breaths. Climbing down, she feels her bones, heavy like waterlogged wood, her blood dense as pressed mud. She returns to the crumbling beast by the parched river. She smooths the dirt around the base of the sculpture, stomps with the flat of her paw. With wild pigs' blood and gray matter and the whites of their eyes, she paints designs of the sun on calm water, and the movements of fish that no longer exist for her to catch. Paints a murder of withered crows in flight. Unhappy with these efforts, she drags her long tail across the dirt and starts over. Paints her father as she remembers him, as the grieving drunken widowed royalty of a mountain forest. She speaks to her dragon father: "You remember me?" she asks. "Because I remember *you*." She tries to explain why she chose art over water, says, "See, I told you. Timid dragons live forever."

She sketches what his response would be: "You can always tell who has no mother." Fei swipes the dirt with her tail once more, paints her *mother* in muscular flight.

Each day, Fei leaves the cave for longer and longer periods. Scrabbles down the mountain. Paints more of her mother, father, the villagers and their angular words, and everyone happily engorged on fatted deer and rabbit. She paints her collection of snakeskins. Tries to paint the anatomy of a cloud, of a home with rolls and ripples, an endless, heaping étage of white water and gray shadow and blue sky.

Each evening, Fei returns to the mountain, hurriedly takes in YingLong's hulking form silhouetted against the moon, and measures his uneven breath. She reminds herself that ghosts do not have shadows. She licks his cheek, tastes salt. She places her snout close to his and inhales deeply his outgoing breath, the smell of swollen river, turbid with silt, the apple dew of summer.

Fei wonders when the end will come, when YingLong's pointy ears will perk for the last time, a gesture not of a final sleep but of him joining other dragons and beasts in his dreams. A frigid gust of wind ruffles her mane. Fei wonders if her dragon of mud and sticks will crack in the deep winter frost, if rodents will harvest the ribbon of hair for their springtime nests, if the elephant skin will dry and crack in the searing summer sun. Will the tears Fei sheds be for YingLong's demise, or for the villagers who will die without rain? What are dreams that fail to take on life and hope? All Fei knows is that she will take YingLong's blood and brain and sclera, and in the darkness paint the sun rising, sun setting. And when the light of the new dawn comes, she will find that she cannot tell the paintings apart.

LINCOLN CHAN: PEAR KING

The San Joaquin and Sacramento Rivers joined on the western edge of California's Central Valley to form the Delta, a collection of slowly sinking tracts of land, islands, and man-made levees. These tracts—dark, peaty soil so full of organic matter that it sometimes caught fire during very hot summers—were perfect for farming asparagus and pears. On nights when he drank too much beer, my father would remind me that I was named after his hero, Lincoln Chan, who was crowned California's Pear King—a title given to the most successful pear farmer in the entire state. *Our sweat feeds the same peat and mud as Lincoln Chan's. I gave you his noble name. What did he do differently that I'm not doing? Why did we not become kings?* Dad would ask in a loud voice. *I bet you didn't know that you were named after royalty. And I bet you didn't know that our family descended from common laborers.* He was referencing my grandfather and great-grandfather, who, in the mid-1880s, tackled a monumental project, working alongside other Chinese immigrants to construct hundreds of miles of peat-block levees on Andrus Island. As I lay in bed, listening to Dad hiccup himself to sleep, I prayed the levee's walls would not break. I dreamed about drowning.

A pear tree in full bloom is a magnificent sight; shrouded in white blossoms, it looks like an enormous silver-haired pear. Mom was shaped like a pear, too. Dad and me, with our wild black hair, resembled the pollinating sticks we used on our trees: slender cigarette holders topped with chicken feathers. While Dad toiled in the winter with our neighbors to build up the levees, adding more peat, straw, and concrete, I spent the chilly months creating a set of pollinating sticks for each of us to use in the spring. I etched my name into the plastic with a hatpin: *Lincoln Chan, Pear King.*

We spent weeks dusting pollen onto millions of pear blossoms in our ten-acre orchard. After years of flagrant pesticide use, there were not enough bees left to do the job, so each spring my family turned into bees.

"Teach me to drive," I said to Flint Wei one afternoon. My eighteen-year-old neighbor had become my best friend three years earlier, after I helped him bury his parents in the town's makeshift cemetery behind the asparagus canneries. They'd been killed in a grisly car accident involving a tractor and a fox. Flint was six foot six, the tallest person I had ever known, the tallest person on the whole island. For extra cash he helped my father in our orchard after working in his own asparagus fields. In the winter and spring, our neighbors pulled together their meager savings and paid him to deliver their asparagus and potatoes to the Stockton, Sacramento, and San Francisco markets.

"You know," Flint said, ignoring my request, "when I leave the island for good, I'll pollinate everything; I'll pollinate the world. I'll find every lonely blossom and use my chicken feathers to join it together with another. I'll be the world's best matchmaker. I'll pollinate pears with apples, peaches with radish, zucchini with watermelon. There are no limits. Every combination is possible. I'll be the world's best worker bee."

This type of proclamation was nothing new for Flint, who was also responsible for taking care of his senile grandmother. Though only two years older than me, he had the determination and patience of a hundred-year-old turtle crossing a highway.

"Come on. Teach me how to drive. You've got a truck, a really cool truck," I said.

"Why would you want to drive? Cars are dangerous."

"I just want to, and Dad won't teach me." I didn't tell Flint that my parents did not want me to drive at all.

"He's just worried about you." Flint dipped a chicken feather into the plastic sandwich bag filled with pollen, reached up his long arm, dusted a blossom, and sneezed. I climbed up to the top branches of the tree, the pollinating stick jammed in the waistband of my pants so I could use both hands. It was early April, but the day had already begun to heat up. I wiped my face with a purple handkerchief. Sweat dripped from my armpits and pooled in my navel.

"What does he have to be worried about?" I touched a feather to a blossom.

Flint studied me for a moment before moving on to the next tree. He was not the kind to bring up my anger issues, and all the things I avoided to keep control: I did not eat spicy foods; I did not drink the beer I stole from my father for Flint; I did not make friends at school because no one, except Flint, was big enough to defend themselves against my rages.

Flint dusted a blossom, then spoke. "Out there, there's all kinds of dangerous things going on." He paused, met my eyes, before continuing, "It's safer here on the island."

But why, I wanted to ask him—why was he always talking about leaving the island? Why couldn't I make it off the island, too? Why did his protectiveness feel like a dismissal? I wanted to tell him that when I wasn't dreaming of drowning, I dreamed of storms pummeling our island, wave upon wave, across the dark fields. As I slept, my bed quilt wrapped hotly around my legs, I dreamed of fire, of jagged rocks and stones. And when I awoke on these nights, Mother would be shaking my shoulder in the darkness, begging me to open my eyes, to stop howling. *Why do you dream in anger? Why? Why so angry?* she would ask each time.

But instead of telling Flint all that, I said, "Whatever. Do you want to come over to watch *Star Wars*? It's on tonight." I climbed back down the tree, swung from its lowest branch.

Flint shook his head.

"Why not?"

"I can't waste my time watching TV."

"What about just lending me your truck? I'll practice by myself."

"No way."

I squinted into the afternoon sun. Flint's black hair, rough like dead twigs and gleaming in the white light, caught in the breeze and lifted off his head. The dust kicked up by nearby tractors and the thick stench of fertilizer were suddenly overwhelming, as if Flint had turned over the earth with his giant hands.

"This is bullshit!" I spat out. I needed to hang onto *something*, so I reached out, grabbed his forearm, and twisted. Flint cursed, snatched up a handful of skin on my stomach, and squeezed. I screamed and let go.

For a while, all he did was glower at me with his back against a tree, rubbing his arm and breathing hard. I rubbed my stomach and glared back. He threw down his bag of pollen and feather stick and walked toward his house with reaching strides. I wanted to blame my outburst on brain biology, youth, hormones, or something that I wasn't responsible for, like cancer or being born with black hair. But I knew that it was something much more selfish.

"What happened to you?" Mom asked in Cantonese that evening, wiping her hands with a dish towel. Approaching our house's front door, I had smelled bacon and bitter greens frying in canola oil, and my mouth watered. I had just finished five solitary hours dusting blossoms and could barely lift my arms.

"Nothing." I kicked off my muddy sneakers and left them by the door, which Mom had painted a good-luck lime green like the rest of our four-room house. I wasn't ready to tell her or anybody what I decided on my slow walk home: If Flint didn't hold a grudge over my outburst, I would do whatever it took to move to Stockton with my best friend and his blind grandma.

"Your dad isn't happy that you take so long. He's so much older than you, looser muscles, weaker arms, but gets more work done. How many trees did you dust today? You talk and talk, cheurng hay, so long-winded. Why ask Flint to help when all you do is talk talk talk? He is tall as a giraffe, his head in the clouds, and still you drag his ears to the ground. What does talk get you? Out of debt? Your own farm?"

I studied my flat, pollen-caked nails. The tops of my hands were sunburned and beginning to spot like my father's.

"Don't scrub your hands too much tonight," Mom said as I walked toward the bathroom. "Maybe if your dad sees the dirt, he won't think he's the only one who's been working."

After a week of my persistence, and an offer to wash his truck for a month of Sundays, Flint agreed to show me how to drive. We took his white Toyota Tacoma, a manual, on the winding levees behind the orchards, and I quickly learned that Flint wasn't very good at teaching.

"Okay, now lift up your foot, nice and slow. Not too fast."

I did it all wrong, lurching from one end of the orchard to the other. I'd get to second gear and then stall. I'd skip the first three gears altogether and grind into fourth. I could tell that Flint wanted to reach over and fix my clumsy movements, but he never did. Instead, he just repeated the same thing over and over. "Lift now! Lift, lift! Why can't you lift?"

I'm not sure who was more frustrated: me, because Flint wanted to practice only for a half hour at a time, or Flint, who could have been working and making money to get off the island. I thought about all of the truck's power in my hands, the speed at the tip of my sneaker. If I got angry enough, I could barrel through the levees and sink my entire island. I wondered if any of the frustrated farmers in the town ever thought of doing that. I wondered how many had tried to leave, and failed.

We lurched through April and May until I could finally make it from first to fourth gear without stalling. While we drove on narrow roads that skirted the island, along crumbling levees and muddy sloughs, Flint told me about his plans for his new life in Stockton.

"I'm going to start my own fish business on Clement Street, near all the Russian videotape stores and Chinese bakeries."

"I thought you wanted to pollinate the world. Anyway, how can you stand the fish smell?"

"I'd run things differently, like the rich white grocery markets. At Whole Foods there are no smells, no flies."

While I maneuvered around tractors and farm workers lunching beside the road, he told me how he hated the smells he carried home with him each night.

"Manure, fermented pear, onion grass. It's like wearing someone else's skin. It's not *me*. When I run my own shop, I'll buy one of those bug zapper lights. I'll have electric fans everywhere, blowing any fish stink out the back door. I'll have windows with screens. My customers will take their time and browse the glass cases with fish and ice under bright clear lights." He sighed happily, absentmindedly tugging on his seatbelt.

The written exam that I took by correspondence after my lessons with Flint was a breeze. Our small town's unofficial "mayor" was the proctor. I only missed two questions, ones anyone would miss. My mom cooked us a big dinner to celebrate. Dad offered Flint a beer. Even though they still did not want me to drive, my parents thought it was important that I win things. Over bowls of rice, steamed asparagus, curried potatoes, and salted pork, I asked Flint in English if he knew what blinking yellow traffic lights meant, or if driving on the shoulder of the road was an okay thing to do—the two questions I'd missed.

He shrugged and said, "If you want to be a driver in the real world, you've got to be ready for the unexpected. With a license, you're showing everyone that you're a fighter. If there's a blinking yellow light, don't just sit there like a turkey, finger in your crack. It's like what Obi-Wan Kenobe says to Luke Skywalker: The force is with you." Flint poured tea for himself without dripping a drop. Mom wouldn't touch her food until I picked up the teapot and served my dad, and then her, before refilling my own cup.

By June, I was ready for my driving test. I walked over to Flint's house after the last day of school so that he could take me to the Stockton DMV, but he hadn't returned from the orchard yet. His blind, eighty-year-old grandmother was working on her handmade pear art in their kitchen. It was a beautiful thing to watch, really. With a knife, she could peel the skin off of kiwis, apples, even ripe plums in one long spiral. She peeled everything this way. She wrapped the skins around a stone that resembled a pear, then let it dry in the sun on the windowsill while she sat and waited for Flint to come home.

When her art was dry, she'd unwrap it, and it would spring back into the shape of a brown, shriveled, lightly sticky, hollow pear. Flint's grandma sometimes mistook me for her grandson, so she'd let me eat the fruit she peeled. She believed the succulent, unmarred insides of fruit were good luck and guaranteed longevity, and she wanted Flint to live forever.

This time I resisted taking the naked apple from her spotted hand, telling her that she should eat it because she was tremendously old. I placed my rolled-up, barely marked DMV written test on the table beside her bowl of rejected fruit peelings.

She shook her head. "There are too many things that you must do in the world, Flint-ah," she said. "And maybe if you eat enough good-luck pear you will not grow up to be a farmer like your parents."

Unlike Flint, I didn't even know why I wanted to leave. I did not have a plan. Everything I did was on impulse, stemming from a need I didn't understand. I wanted to ask her, if Flint's parents were still alive, would Flint still be free to leave? Or would he be stuck like me, chained to his parents' farm? I patted the old woman's arm and accepted her browning apple.

It took two hours to reach the DMV, where Flint and I waited another hour for my examiner. My test began at four sharp, and ended five minutes later.

"Drive forward, over there! Anywhere!" The examiner, a large blond woman with long fake fingernails painted with white daisies, grabbed the window frame as cars barreled toward us on the wide four-lane street. I had no idea where she was pointing. We had stalled straddling the center lane. There were no streets that I could see, just the entrance to a Safeway parking lot. I restarted the engine.

"Now!" She slapped my leg with her palm, and reflexively, I lifted the clutch and jammed on the gas. We shot forward, miraculously making it across the street and into the lot. While I tried to parallel park beside an abandoned shopping cart, the examiner checked boxes on a form, wrote a few messy sentences, then told me that it was time to return to the DMV.

I killed the engine by lifting both feet off the pedals at the same time.

"If I graded drivers like a teacher at a school, you'd get an F. You're just not ready to drive. There isn't even a box to check to describe what you did wrong."

I squeezed my eyes shut, my forehead wrinkling with anger and shame. How would I tell my parents? Or my best friend, who'd wasted hours teaching me to drive?

Later, when I looked at the carbon copy of my test, I saw that she checked the box beside which read *drove over yellow median lines*.

Flint let me drive home. "There was just so much going on, and you didn't get to practice in the city. She should come to Isleton and watch you maneuver around tractors and turtles." He tried to flatten out the thin balled-up sheet with the examiner's notes scrawled on it.

I mimicked the examiner, screwed up my face and made my voice high and whiny. "Don't drive over lines!" Without checking for other cars, I swerved toward the yellow lines in the middle of the road, then back to my lane. The pulpy pear juice I'd drunk for breakfast boiled in my stomach. I wasn't seeing the road anymore, just cracked asphalt, broken reflector dots, grit, gaping potholes, long black rubber scars.

"What the fuck does she know about driving?" I sped through a yellow light.

"Whoa," Flint said as he grabbed hold of the door handle, the examiner's evaluation rolled up in his other hand.

"Why did you even bother?" I asked after we made it out of the city and onto the highway. "You knew that I would fail." My voice grew along with my temper. "You only wanted to teach me because you don't have anyone else who'll listen to you. Everyone is shorter than you, but everyone is your boss. My dad's your boss. My *mom's* your boss. You're just a giant, a freak. A giant freaky loser."

Flint leaned forward to look at my face, but I kept my eyes glued to the road.

"You think I wanted to teach you to drive? You think I want to lose my delivery job to a loser like you? All you do is get mad at people when they're trying to help you. I'm the only one who believes you're not a lunatic."

"I'm not crazy," I said, catching a glimpse of him out the side of my eye. "Your grandmother is crazy."

Flint could have pounded me to a pulp if he wanted to. He was a foot taller than me, strong from hauling fruit, and more determined than anyone I knew. But he didn't need his fists. All he did was speak.

"You need to get off this island. It's either going to kill you, or you are going to kill the island."

I could feel every inch of the road vibrating through the steering wheel. I thought about the bugs smashed against the windshield, the raccoons and rabbits twisted and mutilated on the side of the road. I felt as if I had killed them, every single one of them.

Flint sighed, and I understood that sound. My parents would not leave the Delta until they died, until all that was left of our trees were empty branches.

But Flint would not be like our parents, or a dead tree. He had a choice. I wanted to believe his sigh meant that I had a choice, too. We would find what we needed off of the island. Us together. What name would I carve into my name tag, working in Flint's fish shop? What responsibilities would he entrust me with? Would my anger be enough to drive me off the island; would it drive away my best friend in this new place? I glimpsed Flint out the side of my eye.

"When I can drive," I finally said, "I want to go with you and your grandma."

Flint crossed his arms over his chest, hugging the yellow roll of paper, not caring that it marked how I'd failed. He stared at his lap. A shake of the head at this moment would have been insulting, a sign that he didn't believe in our future. I turned back to the road, but Flint remained stoic and still as a rock.

Flint leaned away from me as I made the turn onto my street. It was twilight; a deep orange glow directly above the trees made it look as if the pear trees were on fire. Flint stared out toward the lighted windows of my house. Mom and Dad were probably in the kitchen, preparing a celebration dinner.

"They make amazing chicken," he said quietly.

"Who? My parents?"

"Yeah, who else, dummy?"

I parked across the road and turned off the engine. We watched the busy silhouettes of my parents moving about the kitchen.

"Do you want to come in?" I asked.

"I should check on Grandma."

"They'll want to thank you. I'm sure they'll give you a medal once they learn I failed the exam."

Flint shook his head and gave a tired laugh. "You don't know what you've got, do you?"

"What've I got? A life picking pears. What kinda life is that?"

"Lincoln. Your parents are really proud of you."

"Doubt it."

"They're your parents. Of course they are."

I tried to imagine my own parents dead and gone, like Flint's. Would I speak of them? Or would I tuck their deaths away, like Flint did, sealing their memories up in sharp metal and sour water, like the asparagus they'd canned? *Orphan* was such a funny word; kids at my school used to call Flint an orphan even though he still had his grandma. In my most jealous moments, when the island felt like it was wrapping its muddy arms around me and squeezing with all its might, I'd tell those kids that Flint wasn't an orphan, that he was independent, liberated. I did not know what he really was, but I wasn't making it up. I knew I was saying something that felt both terrible and necessary. With a guilty shudder, I imagined myself an orphan, finally free of the island, of its narrow, uneven roads, of unreliable fruit and disintegrating levees.

Flint unfolded his long legs and crawled out of the truck. I unbuckled my seatbelt, opened my door, leaving the heavy jangle of Flint's keys on the dashboard. Standing on the road, dirt dusting my sneakers, I felt emptier, my pockets and hands useless without the keys, the steering wheel.

"You know how to drive," said Flint as he got back in on the driver's side. He rested his long arm on the sill, then started the engine. "Say hi to your parents for me, will you?"

The sun had dropped behind the hills in the distance. In the purple-blue twilight, I watched my best friend drive off, dust kicking up behind his tires, his headlights illuminating the road just ahead, reaching into the blackness beyond.

BUG-DOT MILK

I showed Grandma my half-eaten bowl of granola, the many black-and-yellow dots wriggling furiously in the milk. "Ai-ya! Are the bugs swimming?" she said in Cantonese. "Bring me my glasses, Nuan. I like to enlarge everything, you know."

Saturday's late morning light shone through the trees and in the window behind Grandma and made green shadows dance on the kitchen table. Grandma bent her head over the bowl. Her hair stuck out from her bun like pure-white barbed wire. Thick beige socks were bunched up around her ankles like wrinkled elephant skin, and her quilted bathrobe reeked of camphor liniment and dried mushrooms.

"You're lucky they're not worms. Worms would climb up your stomach to eat your brain, make you stupid, and then kill you." Grandma studied me, her head tilted to the side, one eye squinted shut like a pirate's.

"You really ate this?" Grandma dipped a pinky into the milk and tried to get a bug to stick to her finger. "Maybe I should call the granola company and tell them that an eleven-year-old girl almost died from bugs."

My face turned hot. A motorcycle passed by, and its rumblings wrapped around me like a stiff hug. The cereal had been mealy from the first bite, like chewing a wet mouthful of disintegrating crackers that you'd find at the bottom of a sink drain. The taste metallic and earthy and unlike anything I'd ever put into my mouth. I could not tell if the taste was from the bugs or because the granola was exceptionally stale, but I had found myself unable to stop eating even after I'd seen the bugs in my spoon, even after I'd imagined a thousand tiny bugs' excretions dissolving in the milk. And I couldn't explain why I had the urge to rip open the box and pour the rest of it into my mouth. My desire to eat the lively cereal felt the same as when I couldn't stop wiggling a loose baby tooth even though it made my gums bleed and swell.

"You should thank me that I don't call the hospital. Doctors would probably make you drink boiling water."

I could see that Grandma was worked up, so I clamped my lips together and looked her directly in the eyes, the way I was supposed to when I was about to learn a serious lesson.

"Why do you look at me like that? You tell me for weeks to buy this granola because it's the best in world. 'All the kids at school are doing it,' you say. Then a brand new box—so expensive!—is rotten and you eat bug-dot milk."

Grandma began to dial the phone number printed on the granola box. I frowned and looked at my feet. I remembered saying these things. I remembered standing in the cereal aisle at the market and begging Grandma to splurge, to spend money that could have been used for the best cuts of meat or the bigger fish. But I would bite off my own tongue and swallow it before I admitted to Grandma that she was right.

Ten minutes went by while Grandma was on hold with the granola company, and I felt queasy. Questions raced through my mind: Will the bugs eat up my insides? Why did I eat the granola when I saw that it was moving? Why did I tell Grandma?

Grandma looked down into the bowl and spoke, almost as if to the bugs, "When your mom comes home, you tell her you almost died." She clucked her tongue. "Your mom's the smartest. Legal secretary. Very important. But she's never here. Job first, daughter second." She nodded like she was agreeing with something someone else just said.

"You're not supposed to say stuff like that about your own kid," I said, and crossed my arms over my chest. I wished that I were as smart as my mother. Smart people knew how to keep secrets; Mom would never have told Grandma about the bugs.

But in truth, I understood what she meant. I dropped my arms and studied an old scar on my ring finger, remembered the painful slice of the paring knife. I pictured the knobby carrot I'd been practicing whittling on, its rough skin and bright orange insides and sweet shavings that I munched while I waited for Mom to get home from work. Grandma was not yet living with us. Mom had asked why I hadn't bandaged it myself. "Why sit for two hours holding a bloody finger in the air?" I didn't know how to explain why I needed her, why it seemed that bandages applied by someone else always felt better, stuck better, stayed drier, seemed to heal wounds faster. I hated the idea of wrapping my scrapes and cuts before someone else saw them, or could *tsk* with concern for me— if no one saw my wound, then it was like it never happened, my pain was somehow less real or valid.

With the phone pressed up against her ear, one hand covering the receiver, Grandma turned to me. "I was thinking," she began slowly. "Milk is so cold. It goes right into your bones. If I drink milk, I'd probably die from pneumonia. Maybe bugs are not so bad."

For all of her loud talking, Grandma was nervous, I realized.

"Tell me, Nuan, are you happy?" She wanted to know if my stomach hurt.

"I'm okay, Pau Pau."

Grandma's eyes got big, and she waved me over to where she was sitting on the sofa. Someone had finally picked up her call.

"Let me tell you. I buy a brand new box, and something's very wrong," she said in English. She shook the granola box at the telephone receiver to prove she had a box in her hand. "I ask you. I paid good money. Then why do I get bugs in my granola?" She looked up at me and winked, then started to speak in Cantonese, which she did whenever she was excited or angry. "Of course I can prove I purchase it! Didn't you hear me shake the box?" She rolled her eyes. She was dealing with an idiot. "Nuan is too sick to come to the phone. You're lucky my granddaughter's not dead." Grandma's hand holding the telephone was shaking, and her cheeks were red. She used her strongest voice. "I'm telling you now. My daughter is like a lawyer. I call her to do this, do that. My lawyer-daughter is high-priced, working just for me. Anything I want."

I knew that the person on the other end of the line couldn't understand Grandma, and even if he did, he could not know that Grandma wouldn't bother Mom with this. "Lawyers know too many secrets," Grandma would say. "If I am lawyer and know everyone's secrets, my head would explode. No wonder your mom's always nervous." I thought of my dolls, Sushi Bushi and Table Set, which Grandma made for me out of two small pillows stuffed full of rice and decorated with lace and buttons. She'd told me to be gentle with them or they might pop.

She bit her lip as she waited for an answer from the person on the phone. I wanted to shout: Please don't fight her! She is too stubborn, and she will never hang up!

Grandma nodded into the receiver and spelled her name—"S-U-F-A-Y"—and then said slowly, "Su . . . Fay . . . Wong." After giving our address, she hung up, grabbed my arm and jiggled it excitedly. "They're sending us two coupons for free boxes of granola! Free!" she repeated, her eyes bright.

I couldn't tell if the churning in my stomach was from excitement when I pictured getting two more boxes of my strangely delicious, earthy granola or if the bugs were doing laps inside of me. Grandma could hardly contain herself.

"Can you believe what I did? All without your mom's help," she said. "This is the best day."

"Thank you, Pau Pau," I said, smiling.

"Imagine! You ate bugs and did not die, just like I did not give up. You tell me. Is this not wonderful?"

I nodded.

"This will be our secret. Hush hush. If it's our only secret, maybe our heads won't explode." Grandma giggled. She patted my hand, and I helped her stand up.

We poured out the bowl in the kitchen sink. I thought about the dollhouse Grandma built for Sushi Bushi and Table Set out of a discarded refrigerator box pasted with magazine pictures of brand new stoves and leather sofas and a shining grand piano. How warm and colorful and noisy our home had been since she moved in. Grandma hummed the telephone's on-hold music, her hair slipped out of her bun, and her eyes squinted into the sink, looking for bugs. I closed my eyes and held this image of her in my mind.

DUCK HEAD

Mom decides that we'd better hurry because she needs to do some serious cooking, but still she massages each leaf, bulb, and root that she selects from the vegetable stalls, then puts them to her face and breathes in. When I spot a purple potato worthy of being added to our stash, I hold it up for approval. Mom studies it, sniffs it, rubs it between two fingers, and then gives me the head shake. I think about that man in Ohio who brought his spud gun to work. He sat at his desk all day with it, and no one said anything. At closing time, the man shot his boss dead with potatoes. I wonder if the potatoes closed their eyes as they zoomed through the air. I wonder if the ones he used were purple like Mom's, if he took as much care picking them out, and if he washed or cooked them before he loaded his gun. When I ask, Mom says, "If that man cooks his potatoes, he has lunch. Then he is not so angry and maybe eats with his boss instead of kill him."

At the butcher counter, Mom chooses the middle duck. "That is the biggest," she says in Cantonese, jamming her finger against the glass case. "Alix, how big of an egg do you think it once was?" She takes a potato out of her overflowing shopping basket and cradles it like a baby. "I bet you the egg was even bigger than this."

"We already have so much," I say, but Mom shakes her head and uses the potato to knock on the glass. The butcher looks nervous, probably because he knows that Mom will haggle for the best price over anything. Mom likes to brag that the Chinese shopkeepers on Clement Street tell all their butchers, *Ai-ya, watch out for Norma. Hide your biggest ducks if you want to stay in business.*

While we wait in line to pay, Mom tells me about the time she tried to hatch a duck egg with a desk lamp. She was eight years old and living in Shanghai. She'd accidentally cooked the embryo.

"Oh, the smell, it was awful," Mom says, shaking her head, chuckling. "And the ugliest thing I'd ever seen. Totally see-through, it was like a raw shrimp, and its eyes were just these black pinpricks. Your grandpa drank a whole bottle of cooking wine to forget about the odor. Drinking all that made him sneeze for days." She closes her eyes and crosses her arms over her chest. "I wonder why it shook him up so much?"

Mom was not really asking me. This is the thing to remember about Mom's stories: Know them and then you will have something to compare things to if they happen to you; otherwise you'll never figure things out.

As soon as we settle into the house, Mom throws herself into cooking her famous Chinese New Year dinner. It takes hours and hours to pinch off the tips of bean sprouts and sweet peas, dice the fragrant ginger roots, purple potatoes, and daikon, and slice up the stringy gray mushrooms and flat black ones that stink up the house as they soak. Mom washes each bok choy leaf with the care of a surgeon.

At dusk, once the sun slides below the houses and the whole sky turns orange, it is time to set the table. Extra chairs are brought in so that we have nine. I leave a big gap where Grandpa's wheelchair will go.

"I do not feel ready, but the day is already gone," Mom says as she wipes her hands on her apron. Some of her jet-black hair, which has wriggled out of the low bun she always wears when she's cooking, is stuck to the sweat on her cheeks. "Alix, use the special chopsticks for this dinner, the ones that are carved into spirals and painted red."

I nod.

"And put your Grandpa's spot next to my seat."

Mom adjusts her apron strings and then studies her palms like she is inspecting one of my potatoes. I watch her closely, liking the way she moves when she's nervous. In those moments she looks like a little girl, much smaller and quieter than she really is. I notice how dirty and ruddy Mom's hands are compared with the table settings I lay out.

Maybe Mom notices how glossy the chopsticks and ceramic teacups are compared to her hands. Maybe she feels the soreness in her feet from standing in the kitchen all day. Maybe her gesture is a sign of fatigue from years of preparing dozens and dozens of dishes for others, or from how it stopped feeling like a celebration since Dad died, or from the weight of expectation that as the eldest daughter it is her responsibility—but she suddenly declares, "Your grandpa is a no-good, that's what he is when he drinks. He goes crazy and doesn't know what he's saying. I'm putting my foot down. Only tea tonight."

"How do you plan to stop Grandpa from drinking since he always brings his own bottle?"

I must look worried, because she smiles real big. "I will deal with him. Don't stress yourself about this."

"I miss Dad and Grandma."

"Me too. But you know he was no better even when they were still here."

"I know."

"You don't have to sit next to him this year."

"Goody," I say unenthusiastically. "I don't understand why Grandpa gets away with so much. It's not like he's the boss of you."

Mom snorts a laugh. "Ah, my daughter, always using your brain. But he is your grandfather, and you cannot say everything that pops into your head." I wonder if Mom realizes how much I know. I wonder what happens to old stories or memories that we try to forget, and if everything that we think but don't say churns in our brains until it explodes out of our noses, like how broccoli that we eat comes out as stomach gas. Does Mom remember my stories the same way I remember hers?

When my aunties and uncles arrive, the dinner table is crammed with all the dishes Mom has prepared: a purple potato and sweet pea stir-fry, gingery bok choy, braised whole cod, crispy daikon radishes and water chestnuts over rice, and the roasted duck. In the center, I'd placed Mom's monk special, made of garlicky gray and black mushrooms that adorn a steaming pile of clear rice noodles.

"Sit, sit!" Mom commands everyone cheerfully as we gather around the table.

"*Shit* down, everybody," Grandpa mimics. My youngest cousin giggles nervously at Grandpa's swear word, while my aunties frown, though they say nothing.

It is time to dissect the roasted duck. Mom grabs her biggest cleaver, the one with the bamboo handle, and chops the bird in half. Grandpa hungrily licks his lips when the air in the room fills with the scent of roasted garlic. Mom removes the wings and the legs before beginning to slice the breast with a long carving knife. I marvel at how Mom—who has one eye on the duck as she slices and serves the others, and the other eye on Grandpa, watching for the flask in his pocket—does not cut herself. I try to imagine Mom tiptoeing through her childhood. I picture her at eight years old, not tall enough to ride a roller coaster, yet brave enough to creep around in the dark after everyone's gone to bed, searching for the bottles that Grandpa has stashed behind stacks of old telephone books, or behind coffee cans in the pantry, or behind every large piece of furniture in the house. I imagine her crawling out from behind the sofa, dust and spiderwebs clinging to her black hair as she grips a bottle to her chest. She tiptoes to the bathroom. Each night she pours an ounce of vodka down the toilet, and then replaces it with tap water. And each night she prays that his dulled taste buds cannot tell the difference.

"Why does everything you do take so long? You've always been so slow," Grandpa says to Mom.

For a brief moment, the table becomes silent. Mom looks down at her hands, which are covered in oil and flecks of meat. Heat crawls up her cheeks, and at first I'm afraid that she will shout or cry or throw the duck at Grandpa. But then she looks up at me, winks, and I know what she is thinking: brain first, mouth second. She places the carving knife down on the table, then picks up the cleaver, and with a loud *whack*, she chops off the duck's head and presents it to me with two hands, as if she were handing me a royal crown. Grandpa watches, eyes narrowed and arms crossed over his chest as I go for the duck's eyes, dig my tongue into the savory sockets and lick the salty wrinkled hole where its beak used to be.

"A bird's eyes are the biggest part of their head, besides their brain. Did you know that, Alix?" says Mom.

I lick the grease off my fingers.

"If you eat enough of them, you will never need glasses."

I use my fingernails to scrape off the crispy skin, and then set to work on the threadlike tendons and muscles. When I have stripped the duck head mostly clean, I turn it around and around in my hands, then stick the whole thing in my mouth and chomp down with a loud crunch. I think about the man in Venezuala who broke his brain when his angry wife dropped a bushel of sweet potatoes on his head, how doctors drilled a hole in his skull to fix him, but afterward the man didn't know his own name or that he was ever married. I bet if he had eaten his duck head, he would've seen his wife coming from a mile away.

We all start talking at once. My aunties compare parking woes—trying to find a space near our house on Chinese New Year—while my uncles compare who has the bigger appetite. I place the stripped duck head on the edge of my plate so that it faces Grandpa, who stares at it for a minute before moodily picking up his chopsticks and digging into his plate of food. Sometimes you have to show who's the boss.

It grows dark outside, and our chatter softens as we busy ourselves eating. I smile to myself as I think about the long day spent helping prepare the dinner with Mom. One of my cousins throws a mushroom across the table at an uncle. I want the clatter of chopsticks and slurping and chomping to go on forever, and for Grandpa to stay quiet. Mom must read my mind, because she plops another chunk of duck on Grandpa's plate. He starts to complain about the duck head, but a sneeze stops him. I squeeze Mom's hand under the table. She smiles tiredly at me, then turns to study the colorful plates of food; her eyes follow the steam weaving up to the ceiling.

ODONATA AT REST

Bernice Wu pumps her arms as she walks the thirty blocks from her home to Saint Gregory Middle School. Her short black hair bristles in the frigid January sun; her eyeglasses magnify her toffee-brown eyes. Bernice's mind works like that of her mother, a part-time scientist who distributes medication at Golden Gate Senior Care Center. Like a scientist, Bernice uses all of her senses to observe four homeless men her father's age: She notes the pungent odor of urine and liquor, and the fervent sounds of coins rattling in cups. The men count their earnings in public while slurping 7-11 Big Gulps and lamenting their blackened, frostbitten toes.

The men compliment Bernice's green-checkered school uniform, which her mother had ironed that morning, and pose interesting questions as she passes. With one man, Bernice hypothesizes that, yes, tortoises are slower than tarantulas. Bernice drops a coin in his coffee cup; the man recites a singsong blessing about a bum who can still chew gum. Bernice continues on to school, stops to laugh her machine gun *heh-heh-heh* at the faded poster, taped in the greasy window of Yum Yum Dim Sum, of a blond woman eating a slice of pizza.

Bernice's laugh does not endear her to the nuns who run Saint Greg's.

"Today," says Ms. Adams during first period, "I will teach you about the bears and the bees of sex, because you never know what *garbage* you learn out there." The school's youngest nun, who teaches Bernice's favorite subject, biology, sports a blue habit, vermilion pants, and white seashell earrings, and sits on the desktop the way teachers do in movies. "Remember the video about the pack of wild coyotes being born?"

Bernice remembers how her heart had pumped faster and faster as seven glorious pups glided out of the coyote mother's body. Bernice had barely been able to keep her seat; she'd wanted to stand in ovation as the furless pale wet bodies, ears still slicked down, piled on top of each other in the dirt. What a miracle! What pure delight!

"Can you imagine the pain?" Ms. Adams asked the class. "Her body splitting open like that?"

Ripples of uneasy giggles and murmurs filled the classroom. The only two who did not laugh were Bernice and Lamai, a new international student from Thailand, a thoughtful and introverted girl who Bernice had wanted to talk to for weeks, but had been too nervous to.

Ms. Adams moves to the board, draws outlines of reproductive organs and writes their corresponding names. The fallopian tubes connecting the uterus to the ovaries look like legs, and the ovaries remind Bernice of wings. She recalls the tales of her mother's birth, how she emerged as a damselfly—how all of their ancestors could fly, though here in America they are members of a grounded flock.

Bernice has heard stories of her mother's mutation for years. She tries to picture her mother as a damselfly nymph in China, her skin splitting across her back, long translucent wings unfurling, her first wobbly flight. And she imagines her mother's transformation from Odonata into a wingless human, her engorged pregnant belly, wings shorn from her back to be burned along with her medical degrees, the fire filling the house with an enchanted haze fueled by her mother's greatest sacrifices.

But on nights at dinner when it's a struggle to make her mother smile, Bernice wonders why her mother has not reached out to other Odonates—like the elderly Chinese men and women at the nursing home who have told her countless stories about their lives during her rounds. Why doesn't her mother feel lifted by their tales? Why does she not join them at lunch—instead of sitting uncomfortably at the staff table with her terrible manager—and draw inspiration and strength from the elders' decades of experiences?

Bernice makes a sound like a trumpet exhaling. Ms. Adams claps her hands for attention and settles her gaze on Bernice, who is anxious to get to lunch and then next period's computer lab.

Pencils scratch away in notebooks, in what her mother calls *superbly coordinated handedness*. On the chalkboard, Ms. Adams lists three tenets that are practically the school's motto:

1. Take your time.
2. Don't be boy crazy.
3. Don't spend too much money on clothes.

"Are we clear?" Ms. Adams asks the room. "Understand?"

The other girls nod, but Bernice does *not* understand. Why would these be concerns? Her bedroom walls are layered with bright dream-filled art, the periodic table, and posters of Shirley Ann Jackson, Chien-Shiung Wong, and Rachel Carson.

As the other girls rummage in their cubbies in search of sweaters and lunch bags, Bernice thinks of her mother's bedtime stories describing the biochemistry and physiology of horses, stories spoken in Science, the universal dialect of damselflies. She thinks of the tenets her mother taught her: how sexiness is a state of mind, and it is a good mind that knows how to use it; most importantly, that Bernice existed *because* of biology, because different fleshy parts on her parents rubbed together to make sparks, and Bernice grew out of that light. Bernice remembers her pet rabbit giving birth—the smell like salted spongy squid porridge, like a murky morning mouth. She thinks of her mother's skillful rabbit surgery, the ugly red furless skin of the blind kits, how her mother tried to warm the dying doe back to life using a blanket nested inside of her own bed.

Bernice compares her mother's swift-thinking agency at home and as a veterinary surgeon in China to her uninspired work at the senior center doling out heartburn medication. She thinks of the stories her mother tells—of how she hides her intelligence from her arrogant manager, and how she cries in the custodian's closet after a sickly client dies, the tiny utilitarian room becoming a well-stocked cocoon for her tender heart.

Bernice raises her hand and clears her throat like her mother does on the phone with their landlord when the rent is late.

"Yes, Bernice?" Ms. Adams nods.

"My mom says that if you don't use it, you lose it. And it's the *birds* and the bees."

Her classmates' giggles follow Bernice and the nun out into the hallway.

"You hardly speak up in class," says Ms. Adams, "and then you say *this*? What's going on inside that head of yours? Do you want to miss our next field trip to the spider museum because of your attitude?"

Bernice smiles nervously and lets out a weak *heh-heh*.

Ms. Adams frowns. "You got into this school because you won a random district drawing. Do you think you deserve to be here?"

"Yes."

"You're just a kid. What do you know?"

Bernice wants to tell her exactly what she thinks about the inconvenient lottery that landed her in a private school over an hour from home, a school that taught that the Kraken was just a swollen octopus, that space travel was just a symptom of depraved curiosity. A school that promised ivory-glazed Ivy League futures for its students.

But Bernice just smiles at the nun.

"Well, I'm glad you're getting such a kick out of this," says Ms. Adams, her patience shrinking.

Bernice shifts from foot to foot as the nun decides what to do. Everyone knows that spiders' webs can wind around anything that doesn't pay attention; flies that are not observant get caught in the sticky threads and die when the spiders return to drain their blood.

Bernice clicks and unclicks her dental retainer with the flat of her tongue as Ms. Adams calls a colleague on the classroom's beige telephone. The nun nods and mm-hmmms into the mouthpiece and says, "I keep getting these. Mm-hmmm . . . so true . . . I don't know why!"

Ms. Adams's decision is for Bernice to spend lunch break indoors with her. The nun sits cross-legged on her desk while she eats. She shapes her mashed potatoes into God's beard, pours on gravy black as coffee. God looks like he's blistered in the sun because Ms. Adams uses bumpy crumbles of meatloaf for his face. Tangles of green arugula form his long disobedient hair. Bernice unwraps the big soggy bamboo leaf from her tetrahedron-shaped *jung*. She nibbles sweet pork and sticky rice. She slurps her cranberry juice box through a straw and chews on the tips of her disposable chopsticks while Ms. Adams flips through a fashion magazine.

Outside, Bernice's classmates use the lunch break to practice for their Presidential Fitness Award test. From her desk, Bernice watches Lamai struggle to do a pull-up without her wings. The popular girls—blond-haired twin eighth-grade basketball stars—can do all sorts of pull-ups for the president. As Bernice observes her, Lamai dangles from the monkey bars until she slips off. *Thump! Crack! Cry!*

Bernice thinks back to third grade, when she was not yet strong enough to do a pull-up, when she accidentally threw out her retainer with her lunch bag, then sat on her glasses, then her father died, then she refused to leave her bedroom for six weeks, then on the bus she sat on gum, then the senior center manager told her mother that asking for a raise and mentioning her veterinary surgeon degree was "just showing off when you can't even speak perfect English," then a seagull pooped on Bernice's jean jacket *and* her glasses. She remembers the first burning bite of a ghost pepper, tasted on a dare on the same day her mother taught her how to use a microscope and she learned that there were entire universes of biological life teeming inside petri dishes—life so tiny yet so fervent—that there were answers to billions of questions the world might never even know to ask, right under her microscope's lens.

"I dropped out of college to become a photographer for *Vogue*. Did you know that?" Ms. Adams uses her fork to point at Bernice, who shakes her head and listens in fascination for the first time since the coyote video. "I owned expensive cameras. I learned how to outfox bosses, convinced them to hire me over the photographers who'd been there longer. I was building an empire of friendships, like a queen bee and her hive. I had two boyfriends: one Asian, one Italian. I flew all over the world. I was everywhere all of the time, for everyone. I was the opposite of repulsive; I was a magnet."

"How could you give it all up?" Bernice cries out. "Why are you *here*?"

Ms. Adams shrugs and tosses her holy meatloaf in the trash. "I was like you. Independent. Young. Craving . . . everything. But one day on a photo shoot in Seattle, I just didn't want it anymore."

"What, it?"

"Everything."

A vision pops into Bernice's head: an Odonata forced to shed her shimmering veined wings to become a gloomy human mother who steals away to visit the custodian's closet. Bernice marvels at how Ms. Adams could move so freely, how she could shed and then grow new wings wherever she went. Would she, Bernice, turn out like her mother and choose to sit every lunch for the rest of her life with a hundred different Ms. Adamses? Or should she reach out, make friends who understood her, who also drew pictures in their diaries of wings, shimmering blue and green and red and purple?

Ms. Adams stretches out her legs, studies her sturdy leather sandals and flat toenails. "Come, it is almost time for your next class. Clean up. You can go."

"But—!" Bernice throws her arms in the air for emphasis.

Ms. Adams slips from her perch, rests her hand on Bernice's shoulder. "Don't you know what it is that we are trying to teach you?"

"I know."

"What do you know?" The nun's hand drops to her side. "You think that either the world is against you, or that you are the world. Is that right?"

Bernice searches outside the window for her answer. Her class-mates play monkey tag on the bars, undaunted by their full bellies or blistered palms, kicking at each other and howling.

"Out there, there is death. There is disease. But there is also God's love, and there is choice. You can be anything you want to be," says Ms. Adams.

"Mom says the only thing everyone has is . . . we *all* die. It's what we *do*."

"How do you *love?*"

"We have science."

"What does science tell you about love?"

Bernice tries to imagine what her mother would say at home, when she is full of agency and spark, when she rattles off recipes in Chinese like an expert chef, when she recites the periodic table from memory (including the newest elements!) using her specialized Chinese scientific-speak. She remembers tasting her mother's science for the first time, a year after her father died, learning that knowledge can be a source of strength, a new way to understand the world, a new language in which to speak her grief. She imagines the damselfly in free flight, its aerodynamics, its powerful wingbeat, clap and fling. She imagines the dark green stems of a horsetail rush reaching up out of the soggy mud like rigid zombie fingers, and the damselfly's slender perch as it holds its wings over its body at rest.

Bernice takes a breath. "Mom says there are many loves in the world, and the lovers who can't leave them—mushroom lovers, confetti lovers, gin lovers, cheese lovers. Mom says death is evolution. I am evolving. Mom says that we don't all get choices. That when we lost our wings . . . that . . . erm," she stutters. "Mom says—"

"I am telling you." Ms. Adams hands Bernice her backpack. "Life here can be shining and glamorous. And maybe it's just not for *everyone*. Tell your mom that I said so."

Outside, swinging under bars, Bernice's classmates move hand over hand, back and forth, side to side, spinning on their own axes. But Lamai climbs another structure, a glinting geodesic dome: hard plastic, new metal, copper pipe, wood, rope. She reaches the top, lies down on the shape.

Bernice's steps out of the classroom drag into the hallway. They continue to drag on her trek home after school. The straps of her black JanSport backpack dangle off her hips like the tentacles of a sea creature. At the first red light, a nearby bus gives a tired *tssss* as it lowers to release three passengers, two old and one young. There are no homeless to observe. She uses a black marker and draws on a bus stop poster, a walrus—large, loving, long-toothed. At the second red light, Bernice is surprised to see Lamai waiting at the corner.

Perhaps it is the relaxed way Lamai stands, her hands folded before her as if in lazy prayer, that compels Bernice to approach and stand almost close enough to say something to her classmate. She has just opened her mouth to speak when an enormous blue-green beetle lands like a heavy pebble on Lamai's backpack. Bernice marvels at the insect's large armored body. She wonders how it lifts itself in the air, whether beetles have sticky feet that help them crawl up to tall heights before they leap like skydivers, pretending to fly even as they fall. Do their antennae ache as the insects cut through the chilly current, the way that Bernice's teeth ache when she smiles on a cold, blustery day?

Bernice's breath catches when another beetle lands next to the first one. The insects face one another, front legs and antennae waving, as if the beetles are sharing exciting stories about their day. Bernice wishes that her mother was a scuttling overgrown beetle instead of Odonata—confidently carrying her carapace and gossiping with friends wherever she went. As a beetle, she wouldn't need science-speak to armor her. Bernice wonders, though, whether her mother would embrace the rush of a freefall, the sore neck, the icy red blooms on her cheeks as she courageously plunged toward the ground.

Bernice arranges her feet so that they line up with Lamai's; they stand side by side, like friends, for ten red seconds. Cars rush by. The light changes to green. Lamai begins to cross, and Bernice determines she will ask Lamai to join her at the next lunch break, to dig around with her in the schoolyard's dirt, bury acorns or poppy seeds or whatever it is beetles do.

Jogging to catch up with Lamai, who has nearly crossed the street, Bernice laughs as she thinks of how the two of them must look like beetles with their loaded JanSports heaped on their backs. As Bernice runs toward Lamai, arm outstretched to tap her shoulder, her backpack straps lift up in the breeze, trembling like slender black wings.

RADIANCE

Mother cannot bear to throw out books donated to the library under her watch. Stored in our attic: dozens of boxes filled with paperbacks of nearly naked men and women wrestling on the dog-eared covers. At bedtime, Mother models her favorite titles. Tonight, *Lost in Love's Forest*. Mother's arms wrapped around her waist, fingertips digging into her back. Black hair a knotted curtain covering her face.

As my eyelids become heavy, Mother turns out the lights. In the dark, she describes the forest in the background: plush, deep-green moss on moss, and fir trees, pointy stark shadows. The moon, a full-grown star.

It's night all around; my bedroom door ajar to admit light from the bright hallway. The berber carpet glows beneath her mother's feet.

Like many nights before, I wake to Mother and Father arguing through the walls.

Father: "Why do you read her smut?"

Mother: "What's the point of teaching about sex if you don't make it enjoyable? What is light without the flame?"

In my dreams, I paint Father into Mother's paperback forest, reaching down to the fragrant dirt, plunging his fingers deep into termite mounds, then reaching up, dipping fingers in the stars. Fingers tangled in Mother's hair, caressing her earlobes until they glow. Breath and shudders as he leans in, a tree at full bend, moonlight moving on their shoulders.

The next day at school I sweat three hours straight through a secret fever because I don't want to miss a thing. Finally I go to the nurse, who drapes a cool wet cloth on my forehead, plops a bag of ice on my chest. My head throbs, eyes stapled shut. Mother arrives with a thermos of hot apple cider—orange, steaming, spiced with cinnamon. In the checkered hallway, Mother grips my arm, supports my weight. And then: loud roaring. Static and then white space and then static.

And, I'm back.

My first seizure.

On the ride to the hospital, Mother turns the steering wheel with one hand, my sweaty fingers clutched in the other. She whispers promises of savory rice porridge, chicken chunks, boiled eggs with sunny yellow yolks, cherry-red pickled ginger.

Mother: gentle, hopeful, a balm.

Me: wanting to be sick forever.

Seizures make you famous with your friends. Back at school, they ask: Are seizures like earthquakes? Does it hurt? Do you get dizzy from all that shaking?

Fame makes me flush, a lit flame.

Bell Jian, fellow fourth grader and my neighbor, not quite a friend but not a stranger. A foot taller than me, with hair full of static. Mother calls her Mountain. Everyone knows that her grandmother can't feed or bathe herself, that Bell pushes the old woman in a wheelchair up and down our street, both of them silent and creeping as ghosts. She stutters an *um* when she is nervous.

"Can you, *um*, help me do it?" she asks.

"You can't just make someone seize."

"Where do you go when you seize?"

My first seizure I did not travel far. I did not know where to go. By my third, fourth, I got the hang of things. In my seizures, I'd tell the other kids, I've sparred with green giants. I met people lost in their dream worlds, and gave them high fives as they returned to waking. In my seizures, I was left-handed, but I bowled with my right. In my seizures, all the extinct animals were alive, saber-toothed tigers and dinosaurs and mammoths just roaming around looking for what's good to eat.

"Dad, um, says it's like dying."

"It is and it isn't," I say with a mysterious smile, the kind that indicates I have more to say but I won't.

"I want to know where you go when you die."

"You're crazy."

Mountain's face crumples.

In truth, I'm afraid to tell her that if I had the power to see a seizure coming, I'd run away as fast as I could. I don't choose to seize. I am not brave enough to purposefully travel to a place I can't remember, a place not on a map, a place I might never come back from. Why would anyone want that?

"You've never lost someone you love," she says as she turns to walk away. I know she is worried about her grandmother. "You don't know how it feels."

That night, Mother models a farm scene. Cows mooing in tandem, sensual pink udders, dense black-splotched coats. Father knocks on their bedroom wall with his fist, says loudly through the ripped, rose-print wallpaper, "Where's *our* love story?"

"We have a *twenty-year* love story!" Mother's lips press to the largest flower. She chuckles at her own cleverness.

We watch the sheer curtains billow in the night breeze, the window breathing in and out, the luminescent moon.

"Have you heard about how the moon shares our earthshine?" Mother describes the difference between *libido* and *albedo*. Make and be. Love and light. "Libido. You *make* love. That will come later. Albedo, you *be* love. Now, always. Both have their own resonances and heat, tides and currents. When the day comes that you are ready to *make* . . . it's like . . . it's like the first time you took a step, or memorized your first phone number, or spelled your name. Do you remember that feeling? When all of a sudden the funny shapes drawn and strung together on a piece of paper meant something, when the squiggles and lines and dots became *you*? It is you, but it isn't. Now you exist on a piece of paper *and* out here, sitting at the desk with the pencil in your hand."

I shiver as I remember the feeling, the sense of displacement, the excitement and thrill of writing myself onto the page. Like seizures. Here and not here. You want to. You don't want to.

Mom must see the concern etched in my face because she pats my hand. "Don't worry about it right now. Okay? One day it'll all make more sense."

I ask about seizing—the same question I ask each night. "Will I always be this way? What if I don't come back?"

"Have you heard the one about the girl who could lift a cow?"

I shake my head. I tell Mother how Bell had asked at recess, then at lunch, "Please. Can you help me, *um*, do it? Help me do it. Please." How, when I saw her in the bathroom after school—gritty, powdered yellow soap scraping between her palms—she'd shorthanded to just, "Please." How *please* became Bell's *um*.

Mother responds, "Girl lifts a baby calf when it's small, spotted and furry, size of a middle-aged Cocker Spaniel. Each day she lifts the calf. And each day, the animal gets bigger. Size of a bigger dog, then a gangly emu, then a majestic mountain lion. Then one day it's a full-grown cow that Girl, arms trembling under its great weight, lifts straight overhead. You can do anything you put your mind to. You can turn off the moon by just closing your eyes."

The next day, I watch fifth-grade boys, warped by sugar and boredom, playing Guantanamo in the schoolyard. Rich boy, Tuff Lee, dumps orange soda on a third grader, pulls the soaked t-shirt halfway over the poor boy's head, binding his arms and face in the fabric. By the time a teacher reaches them, the third grader has blacked out.

Bell is not at school, some kid says when I ask, because she needed to be at her grandmother's funeral.

In Bell's backyard, it's stifling even in the shade of her apple tree. Fruit in abundance, sunburnt nickel-sized circles on top of red skin. Me, barefoot, in a tank top, naked shoulders. I tell Bell to crouch down. "*Good.* Now, squeeze your elbows in."

Bell, sweating in all black, in a duck-and-cover position. She looks up. "You sure this is what a dying person's like?" Behind her, magenta bougainvillea shrouds a screen door, the back of her green house faded to yellow.

I throw Bell my biggest orange-peel smile. That look. "I'm sure! Hold your breath. Okay, squeeze everything in. Really *squeeze!* Don't poop your pants."

"What if I die?" Bell's whole body is shaking. A leaf in her electric hair, bark crumbling onto her back. Bees murmur overhead. Apple pulp mashes between my toes. I think of Mother's dog-eared novels, splayed open on her chest as she sleeps. The trembling cow udders. The spent moon. And Father's mouth roaring, hot static yelling, fingers squeezing Mother's earlobes.

"Get real tight. Hold your breath. Cut all oxygen to your boobs. Shut down your brain. Can you feel it? Man, this is so bad for you. . . . Good! Hold it. Hold it. . . . Now STAND!"

Bell springs to standing. I hold her against the tree, press into her chest with both palms, all my weight. Bell's eyebrows stitch with hurt. She blacks out, crumples to the ground.

She lies there.

And lies there.

How will she come back? Full of love and moonlight? Where she went, is it full of ghosts sitting together on clouds, shoulder to shoulder, legs dangling over the velvety white edges, busy with gossip—their excited whispers and greetings of old friends filling the air with white noise, like the roaring, flickering snow on old-fashioned televisions that have lost their tuning? Where she went, would she find her grandma in the ghostly throng, would she be able to hear the old woman call out to her through all the static?

I place a hand on Bell's forehead, feeling for life. Bell suddenly pops up, and I, caught by surprise, slap her in the face. She rubs her cheek, red and steaming, smiling. Pure radiance. I drop to my knees, take her by the shoulders and shake until her teeth chatter. "Well? What did you see? Tell me! Tell me! What did you see?"

ACKNOWLEDGMENTS

I'd like to thank my phenomenal editor at Acre Books, Nicola Mason, for nourishing my stories with her deeply insightful questions, comments, intuition, and humor. I'm so thankful for her patience, her copy-editing expertise, her guidance with exploring my characters' true desires, and for helping me to grow as a writer. I'd like to thank both Barbara Bourgoyne (for her marvelous book cover and typesetting design) and Monica Canilao (whose breathtaking paper quilt is featured on this cover) for giving my stories such a beautiful a home within their incredible art.

I am indebted to all my amazing friends, classmates, workshop-mates, colleagues, teachers, and mentors—at San Francisco State University (SFSU), North Bay Writers Group, Writing Rainbow, The Escapery, Wayward Writers, Mission Pie Writing Group. I'm so thankful for these beautiful creative spaces that encouraged and inspired me, held space for my contemplations about my heritage and queerness, and that were instrumental in helping me to write the stories for this book. And I want to thank Why There Are Words, Litcrawl, Hazel Reading Series, Saturday Night Special, Lyrics & Dirges, InsideStorytime, Nomadic Press, RADAR, Voz Sin

Tinta, and all of the phenomenal Bay Area literary reading series that provided such loving spaces for me to share my words, to stretch my voice. I am so thankful for the extraordinary editors at all the literary journals who took a chance on me by publishing my work, who helped me with shaping these stories, who championed my work and the work of so many artists.

I truly wish that I had the space here to thank *everyone* who helped me to complete this book through their generous workshop feedback, or through their editorial expertise, or through reading early drafts of the manuscript despite their demanding schedules, or whose brilliant questions motivated me to dig deeper and to work harder to elevate my craft. In this short space, I will begin with: Adam Zane Cook, Adam Manfredi, Adrian Ibarra, Ai Ebashi, Arisa White, Aurelia Cortez Peyron, Barbara Solomon, Beverly Morrison, Blossom Plumb, Celeste Chan, Chad Koch, Christopher Allen, Chris Fink, Chris Tusa, Conrad Panganiban, Courtney Miller Santo, Dan Schifrin, Daniel Suarez, Deni Li, Diana Fisher, Diane Glazman, Gloria Jorgensen, Ellen Parker, Esther Patterson, Evelyn Aikman, Flavia Stefani Resende, Gen Del Rey, Haldane King, Heidi Van Horn, James Warner, Jane McDermott, Jared Roehrig, Jason Mendez, Jen Kulbeck, Jennifer Barone, Jennifer S. Cheng, Jennifer Lewis, Jenny Alton, Joe Ponepinto, John Haggerty, John Philipp, Joseph O'Brien, Juliana Delgado Lopera, Kalpana Mohan, Kar Johnson, Katelyn Keating, Kathryn Kruse, Kay Unlanday Barrett, Kayle Frayre, Keith Donnell, Kelly Sandoval, Kendra Schynert, Kendra Vanderlip, Kimberly Gomes, Lauren O'Neal, Lisa Ampleman, Luke Dani Blue, Maia Ipp, Margaret Spilman, Mark Budman, Matt Borondy, Matt Carney, Maxine Chernoff, May-Lee Chai, Melissa Ladrech, Miah Jeffra, Muriel Leung, Nara Dahlbacka, Patricia Reynoso, Philip Harris, Phillip Barron, Ploi Pirapokin, Rachel Kessinger, Ramon Shawntez Jackson, Rene Vaz, Renee Hamlin, Roxanne Villaluz, Sam Rigel Bowman, Sara Marinelli,

Sarah Heady, Sasha Wright, Shannon Peavey, Shasta Grant Huntington, Sherrel McLafferty, Shinjini Bhattacharjee, Sommer Schafer, Stacey Matthews-Winn, Stephanie Doeing Nicoletti, Stephen Langlois, Steven Wilson, Susan Keller, Tara Laskowski, Terry Boero, Tomas Moniz, Traci Chee, Val Gryphin, Vivian Underhill, Wendi Olson, Yume Kim. . . .

I'd like to thank my friend, Carson Beker for teaching me, through their art and friendship, about lionheartedness. And I am so thankful for sharing a cabin for two weeks with Carson (and a dead bird, a startled apple-eating deer, and three hundred pounds of cheese), where they gave me the courage to write the title story for this collection. I am so thankful to my very first creative writing teacher and mentor, the wonderful Peg Alford Pursell, for her brilliant teachings, for helping me find my voice, and for always believing in me. And I'm so thankful to Carolina De Robertis, for her extraordinary mentorship, guidance, and support with every part of this book. I'm so thankful to all of my brilliant teachers at SFSU—Nona Caspers, Barbara Tomash, Michelle Carter, Toni Mirosevich, Anne Galjour, Andrew Joron, Dodie Bellamy—who cultivated such dynamic and supportive learning spaces and such brilliant curricula that inspired me to write many of these stories.

And, I want to thank my lifelong love-bug and best friend, Matthew "Bug" Cover, for sharing his incredible Science and bugs, for believing in me, for supporting my art every step of the way, and for loving me with the biggest and most patient heart in the world. I want to thank the sweetest doggy in the whole world, Luna, for our long hikes together and for her biscuit smells and white stripe and soft ears. And I want to thank my entire family: all my amazing aunties and uncles and cousins and in-laws, and my beautiful siblings and "sig figs"—Lauren and Justin, Becky and Chris, Steven and Daphne—for their endless kindness and love.

*   *   *

Stories in this volume earlier appeared (sometimes in altered form) in the following publications: "The Richmond" in *Catapult*; "Wearing My Skin" in *The Pinch*; "Spider Love Song" in *Tahoma Literary Review*; "How to Become Your Own Odyssey, or The Land of Indigestion" as "I See It All" in *Gone Lawn*; "Louise" in *FRiGG*; "She Is a Battleground" in *Lunch Ticket*; "The Fox Spirit" in *Hermeneutic Chaos Journal*; "Lincoln Chan: Pear King" in *Beloit Fiction Journal*; "Anatomy of a Cloud" in *Typehouse Literary Magazine*; "The Unfed" in *Flapperhouse*; "This Is Me" in *Foglifter*; "Odonata at Rest" in *Liminal Stories*; "Radiance" in *Fiction Southeast*; "Mom's Desert" in *Identity Theory*; "Bug-Dot Milk" in *Prick of the Spindle*; and "Duck Head" in *Mill Valley Library Literary Review*.